Vertical Reflexology

A revolutionary five-minute technique to transform your health

Lynne Booth

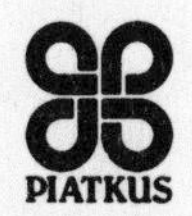

To Adam and Alice

VRT does not replace normal allopathic medical treatment. It is a means of supporting and complementing such medical treatment. If you have any acute or chronic disease you should seek medical attention from a qualified medical doctor. The author and publisher accept no liability for damage of any nature resulting directly or indirectly from the application or use of information in this book.

Published in 2000 by
Judy Piatkus (Publishers) Limited
5 Windmill Street
London W1T 2JA
e-mail: *info@piatkus.co.uk*
Reprinted 2001

For the latest news and information on all our titles,visit our website at www.piatkus.co.uk

A catalogue record for this book is available from the British Library
ISBN 0 7499 2132 3

Designed by Jerry Goldie

Illustrated by Lesley Wakerley
Data manipulation by
Phoenix Photosetting, Chatham, Kent
Printed and bound in Great Britain by
Butler & Tanner Ltd, Frome

Contents

Acknowledgements

My parents, brothers and sister for their love, support and many contributions to my work. My colleagues, Barbara Stanhope-Williamson, Alison Dobbins and Hedwige Dirkx for their invaluable advice, reflexology skills and loyalty. Anthony Porter for his inspiration, belief in VRT from its earliest days and for teaching me reflexology in the first place. Huon and Fran Hassall in Australia for their interest, dedication and expert advice. Dr Virginia Royston for her friendship and help in checking the medical aspects of the book. Graham Purches for his journalistic advice and interest in the book from the very beginning, Kathryn Marsden for re-introducing me to the value of reflexology and nutrition many years ago and to Kathleen Collings, R.G.N. for enabling me to research VRT and conduct a medical trial. My friends, clients, fellow reflexologists and nursing home residents for their unfailing co-operation, enthusiasm and willingness over the years to be part of my Vertical Reflex Therapy research.

Finally, my husband Adam and daughter Alice for their amazing patience, love, tolerance, humour, help and encouragement during the writing of this book.

Foreword

For many years I have been an enthusiastic devotee of reflexology and can testify to its healing qualities. I incorporated it into my nutrition practice over a decade ago and never ceased to be amazed at how many people found it so beneficial. It was during my tenure as a practitioner that I first met Lynne Booth.

Lynne has spent many years developing the unique therapy that is described so beautifully in this book. Vertical Reflex Therapy (VRT) is a new and advanced technique that can be used either in conjunction with traditional reflexology or as a powerful procedure in its own right. But what makes it so special and so different?

Reflexology is traditionally practised when the body is in the prone – horizontal – position. For most people, lying down and 'having your feet done' is a wonderfully restoring experience. No-one – before Lynne – has ever researched the important differences and effects that can occur when the foot is weight-bearing or how much additional benefit there is to be had when these new and potentially deeper reflexes are taken into account. This is not to deny the incredible results that can be had from conventional reflexology – but feedback from practitioners and patients who have experienced both methods strongly suggests that the body tunes in to additional healing powers when VRT is used. And from a purely practical point of view, there are many instances when it can be easier to treat someone who is standing or sitting, rather than lying down, for example if the patient is not so mobile or where time is limited; VRT can be given successfully in only a few minutes.

Lynne Booth's dedication and exceptional hard work has already been of benefit to many many people and of particular help to the elderly, the disabled and to babies and children. Not only has there been a huge groundswell of interest from the general public in her innovative methods but also from practitioners wanting to learn more. Of obvious value as an adjunct to existing professional skills, VRT is also safe and straightforward enough to use at home, for friends and family; an advanced tool for reflexologists but accessible and effective, in its simplest form, to anyone willing to learn the basic technique.

In addition to bringing her dedicated research and practising skills to VRT, Lynne Booth has also achieved something else that is, I believe, extremely special and very important. Her professional approach and dedicated research has triggered a genuine interest in VRT from the medical profession, not only emphasising to them the known benefits of traditional reflexology but demonstrating the unique and drug-free approach that is VRT. Only with integration and understanding between orthodox medicine and the less invasive but powerful natural therapies will healing become truly complementary.

Lynne Booth is an exceptional lady with outstanding curriculum vitae as a real human being and a talented teacher and practitioner. I wish her every success with the launch of *Vertical Reflexology*. Learn from her. You won't regret it.

Kathryn

Kathryn Marsden

Kathryn Marsden is a nutritionist, columnist, lecturer and bestselling author. She writes regularly for leading magazines and the national press, teaches in adult education and has written twelve books on nutrition and holistic health.

Introduction

SOME OF THE BEST DISCOVERIES HAVE BEEN MADE BY CHANCE. A WELL-KNOWN example is Newton's formulation of the law of gravity, which is reputed to have come about as the result of an apple falling on his head. In my own case, to a far less ground-breaking extent, some good fortune and intuition, coupled with research, surrounded the eventual discovery of Vertical Reflex Therapy.

Back in my student days in the late 1970s complementary therapies were proliferating madly. A flatmate had a summer job at the BBC where one of his colleagues, who had learnt reflexology, would work on the many willing pairs of feet in the studio. I was fascinated to hear about it, and became an eager guinea pig for this new therapy.

Reflexology, as many readers will already know, involves working on various pressure, or reflex, points in the feet which relate to different parts of the body. Our feet, with their twenty-six bones in each, are an amazing piece of engineering. Narrow ankles bear our weight throughout our lives, if we are fortunate, and are one of our principal means of balance. In the modern world we pay scant regard to this area of our anatomy, but in ancient Egypt physicians greatly respected the feet and regarded them as one of the key 'windows to the body'. The tomb of the physician Ankhmahor at Saqqara contains wall carvings which illustrate the seven healing arts of mankind: among them is a depiction of foot and hand reflexology being practised.

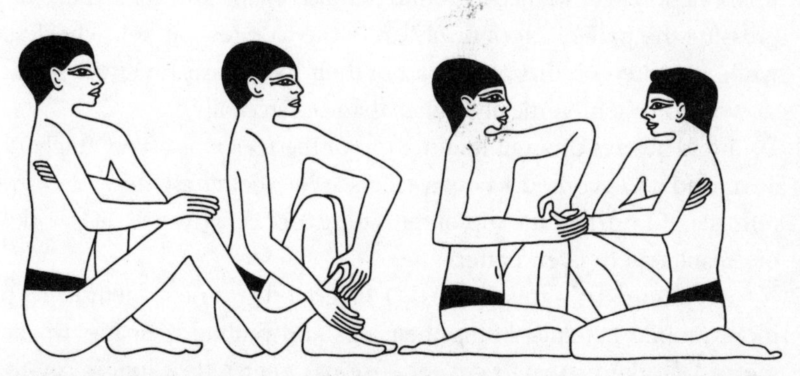

Egyptian reflexology scene (2300BC) on the tomb wall of Ankhmahor, the royal physician at Saqqara. The patient says, 'Don't hurt me'. The practitioner replies, 'I shall act so you praise me'.

Although my interest remained, it was not until 1990, when nutritionist Kathryn Marsden re-introduced me to this 'brilliant hands-on therapy', that I was finally able to devote some time to learning how to treat people with this centuries-old therapy. After my first local evening class I came home thrilled with what I had discovered and anxious to experiment with my new-found knowledge. When my husband complained about the after-effects of a heavy business lunch I amateurishly set to work on his feet, prodding them uncertainly and making constant references to my charts. Within a few minutes his stomach and diaphragm felt more comfortable, and half an hour later all pain and discomfort had gone. It was not surprising, then, that he encouraged me to go ahead and find the best possible teaching!

After training at the International Institute of Reflexology in London, I worked in a clinic and a hospital before concentrating on my private practice. Then I was asked to hold a weekly clinic at a large residential nursing home in Bristol. I have worked there ever since, treating elderly and chronically sick people with rewarding, and sometimes spectacular, results. It is the residents whom I have to thank for enabling me to discover and develop Vertical Reflex Therapy, which now benefits people of all ages.

In traditional reflexology patients are treated while lying down, but when working with wheelchair patients this was not an option for me. Indeed, it was often not possible to work on the sole of the foot at all – by the time I had got a paralysed leg out of a caliper or tried to lift a swollen or heavy foot I was straining my hands, and often found myself at too difficult an angle to access the sole of the foot properly. Adapting to circumstances, I found I could obtain excellent results from pressing the patient's foot firmly on to the foot rest of their wheelchair while I worked on the upper part of their foot. I was, in effect, starting to work on them vertically rather than horizontally.

I had always thought that the top of the foot was a very uncharted area, and as I worked I began to discover seemingly new or deeper reflexes. If I pushed the top of the sitting foot downwards as I worked, the results were even better.

Encouraged by this success, I extended my new method to my more mobile patients, lifting their legs and pulling their feet towards me as I worked so as to create tension. Other reflexologists say they too have instinctively performed this 'pulling' technique: by doing so, they feel they can get more deeply into the hip/pelvic reflexes.

Further training, including Anthony Porter's excellent Advanced Reflexology Training (ART) courses, enhanced my work and improved my skills. However, I was still not able to work out how to gain deeper access to the new reflexes I was finding on the feet that were resting on wheelchair foot supports. I felt intuitively that I had hit on something unusual when I successfully treated patients whose doctors had said they could do no more for them. The missing piece of the jigsaw finally appeared in the guise of a frail old lady who had been involved in a minor accident at the nursing home.

Dorrie, who already suffered from osteoarthritis and osteoporosis and could walk only with a stick, had injured her hip a few days earlier when she was struck by a fellow-resident's electric wheelchair. I was late for my weekly clinic when I came across her, so I quickly knelt down and administered some on-the-spot 'first aid'. While she remained standing, I worked the hip, leg, spine and pelvic reflexes around her ankles for no more than ninety seconds.

A delighted Dorrie telephoned me later to say that a mere ten minutes after I had gone she was experiencing pain and warmth in her injured hip, followed by soreness and tingling. The pain had quickly worn off, however, and by the following morning she could lift her foot some way off the ground. This improvement was accompanied by greater mobility than she had known for months. I immediately realised that *weight-bearing* was the key to faster results from reflexology – and what better way to achieve that than by standing? Vertical Reflex Therapy was born!

After a series of short treatments combining conventional reflexology and VRT, within seven weeks Dorrie had cast off her walking frame in favour of a stick. In ten weeks she had begun climbing stairs and travelling on buses, and claimed she felt in better shape than before her accident. Five years on, she is still virtually pain-free and mobile despite an original prognosis of being wheelchair-bound within eighteen months.

As soon as I saw the rapid improvement in Dorrie's condition I began to put all my knowledge, hunches and past research into practice. At the end of their standard reflexology treatments, I asked my regular clients if I could experiment on their skeletal reflexes in a standing position. Thirty-eight-year-old Helen was one of the first. A businesswoman who had to drive long distances in the course of her work, she had experienced pain in her left leg since injuring her hip on a waterslide at a sports centre. After I had worked on her hip/pelvic reflexes in the ankle area while she remained standing, she commented that it felt more painful than when she was lying down. But a week later she called me to say that she had driven several hundred miles without a twinge of pain, and had remained pain-free.

In the early months when I was using the new treatment I was concerned that some of my clients, whose hip and knee joints had degenerative disease and were surrounded by wasted muscles, might overdo things. But this simply does not happen, and it is clear that some form of regeneration must be taking place. Scores of people who have been treated with VRT since the mid-1990s are being constantly monitored: they are walking, climbing stairs and making the most of their second chance of an active life with no repercussions.

Soon VRT had been shown to treat not just the familiar orthopaedic problem areas of backs, hips and necks, but other conditions including asthma, period pains, irritable bowel and ME (myalgic encephalomyelitis). In theory, any condition can be helped and anyone can be taught to use VRT in its most basic form. The only rule is to work for a maximum of five minutes at any one time, since the therapy is so powerful.

This book is a practical guide for both professional reflexologists and newcomers to the technique who would like to treat friends and family. It will show you how to gain or give others the same benefits as Dorrie, Helen and so many others. Reflexology has been around for nearly five thousand years, and would have disappeared long ago if it had been ineffective; indeed, medical trials are now beginning to prove its efficacy. And VRT is simply another step forward in the fine-tuning of this wonderful, non-invasive therapy. When his painful frozen shoulder freed up after a single VRT treatment one client said to me, 'I don't care how it works – I just know it *does* work!' It can work for you too.

'Since reflexology is a professional therapy requiring intensive training in anatomy, physiology, theory and techniques, surely VRT should be taught only to qualified reflexologists?'

My strong belief is that this simple but powerful therapy should be shared with as many people as possible. VRT in its most basic form is extremely easy for virtually anyone to learn and apply, but is still very effective. However, only qualified reflexologists are eligible to attend VRT training workshops, as these techniques were developed to enhance conventional reflexology. For professional practitioners, this book offers a number of advanced techniques and methods of treatment.

An overview of reflexology

The principles behind reflexology

Restoring balance, reducing stress

DESPITE ITS EFFECTIVENESS AT TREATING A VAST RANGE OF ILLNESSES AND INJURIES, reflexology does not set out to heal specific ailments. Rather, its aim is to produce in the body a state of relaxation and *homeostasis*, a Greek word meaning balance. Our bodies are equipped with wonderful self-healing facilities, but these often fail to work properly because the vital energy pathways are blocked due to degeneration and the stresses and strains of life. Reflexology redresses that situation by reducing stress, accelerating the repair work done by the body and boosting the immune system.

The theory behind reflexology is that the tension, congestion and possible disease in the body are mirrored in the feet and hands. Each foot and hand represent one half of the body, and the charts on pages 71–77 show the corresponding reflex for every part of the body. Reflexologists do not diagnose specific conditions; but if a particular reflex is tender or feels granular when pressed, it indicates that the corresponding body area is in need of stimulation to boost its natural healing powers.

Since it treats the entire person, not just the symptoms, reflexology is a holistic therapy. Its appeal has been universal and lasting because:

Reflexology in brief

- Reflexologists do not prescribe, diagnose or treat specific illnesses, but work on the body to stimulate its own healing response.
- Reflexologists are trained to work various reflexes to help certain conditions.
- Reflexology and VRT can be used on their own, with other therapies or alongside mainstream medical care.
- Reflexology is for healthy as well as sick people, for young as well as old.

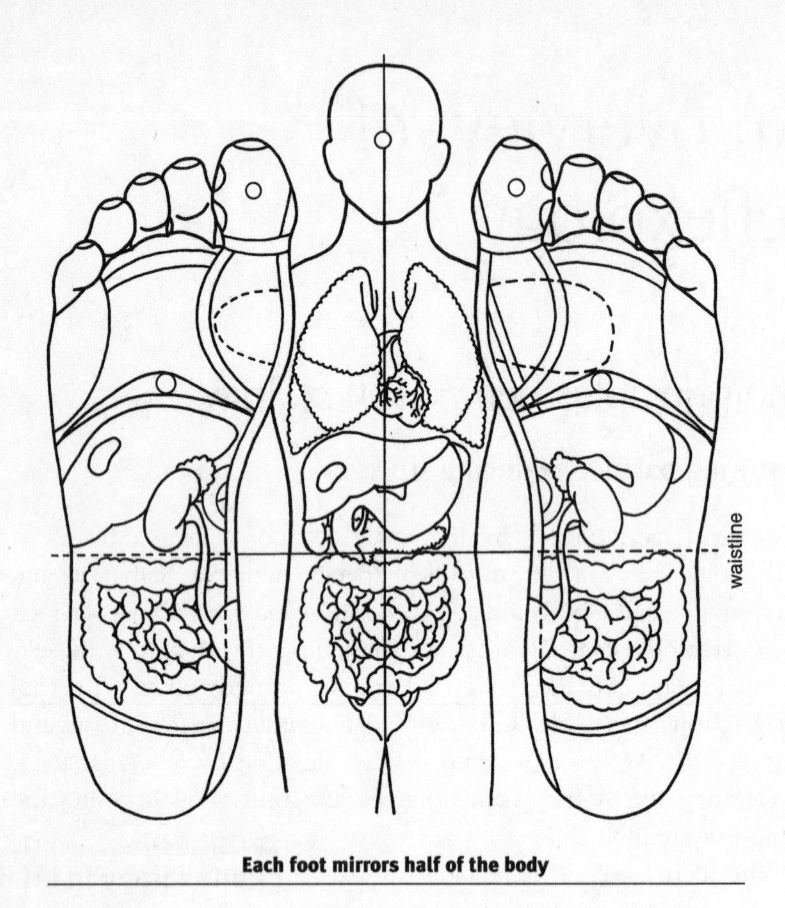

Each foot mirrors half of the body

- it is an all-encompassing treatment, since all the organs, the glands and the skeletal system can be accessed and stimulated through the feet and hands.
- it is very user-friendly as it is non-invasive (unlike surgery, for instance), the clothes do not have to be removed, and the feet and hands can be accessed easily anywhere, at any time.

Self-help

The self-help aspect of reflexology is very important. A few minutes a day spent working on your own hands or feet can be an important part of taking responsibility for your own well-being. Self-help treatment is especially useful if you are having professional treatments, as it can accelerate the natural healing processes in between sessions.

An ancient history

Reflexology to restore a body to a healthy balance has a history spanning five thousand years. The ancient Egyptians have already been mentioned, and traditional Chinese medicine has for centuries used the feet to stimulate reflexes as well as using acupuncture to balance the meridians. In its ancient form, reflexology was possibly introduced to Europe after Marco Polo opened up the silk routes from China in the thirteenth century. It is ironical that some cynics speak of therapies such as reflexology, acupuncture and herbalism as 'new age' treatments.

In the early twentieth century reflexology reached the USA. An ear, nose and throat surgeon named Dr William Fitzgerald used a technique called Zone Therapy to help anaesthetise patients during operations. Dr Edwin Bowers helped map out points on the hands and feet that corresponded to different areas of the body. In 1915 he published an article called 'To stop that toothache, squeeze your toe!', followed by a book entitled *Zone Therapy or Curing Pain and Disease*.

A physiotherapist called Eunice Ingham became interested in Zone Therapy in the early 1930s when working as an assistant to Dr Jo Shelby Riley. Dr Riley had used the technique for many years, but it was Ingham who really spread the message: her work in developing modern Zone Therapy and mapping out the feet was so influential that she became known as the Mother of Reflexology. This intrepid and forthright woman travelled across America for some thirty years, teaching reflexology first to nurses and doctors and then to non-medical practitioners. She renamed the technique, developed the charts and theories that form the basis of modern teaching, took reflexology out of its medical context and established it as a major complementary therapy. In 1952 her nephew, Dwight Byers, founded the International Institute of Reflexology, which has since trained thousands of professional reflexologists around the world.

Enlightened employers

In Denmark, reflexology is the leading complementary therapy. Over a quarter of the population have tried it, and most have reported good results. After Danish Airlines and the Danish Post Office began providing reflexology services for their staff, they recovered more rapidly from muscular/skeletal conditions and took fewer days off work through sickness.

A complementary therapy

Towards the end of the twentieth century reflexology began to achieve recognition as a distinguished complementary therapy with an important role to play in hospitals, clinics and private practice throughout the world. The word 'complementary' as used here means that it complements conventional medicine, and many reflexologists work alongside doctors and nurses in hospitals and hospices.

Reflexology and other therapies also complement natural health care. This means that anyone who eats nutritious food, exercises regularly and makes time for relaxation can enhance their general health by stimulating the body through reflexology, acupuncture or aromatherapy, for example.

What a reflexologist sees in feet

A mini-map of the body

The concept of points on the feet mirroring areas of the body is easier to understand and learn than, say, the principles of acupuncture, in which meridian lines and points cover the entire body. The foot reflexes form a miniature map of the body, starting with the head, brain and sinus points on the toes and moving downwards to the pad of the foot which contains the shoulder, arm and chest reflexes. Each foot represents half of the body, so although there are kidney and spinal reflexes on both feet, there is a heart reflex mainly on the left foot and a liver reflex only on the right.

To make life easier for the reflexologist the foot is divided into sections (see opposite). If you are new to reflexology and want to learn the Revitaliser treatment you can bypass learning about the individual reflexes. Instead you can work on the feet as described on p. 23, which will automatically provide a holistic treatment and stimulate the entire body.

Sensitivity

There are over seven thousand nerve endings in each foot. The feet are far more sensitive than the hands because they are not exposed to as much contact, pressure, movement and lifting (although the hands are equally responsive to reflexology). Contrary to some people's fears, reflexology does not make you feel ticklish: the techniques should be

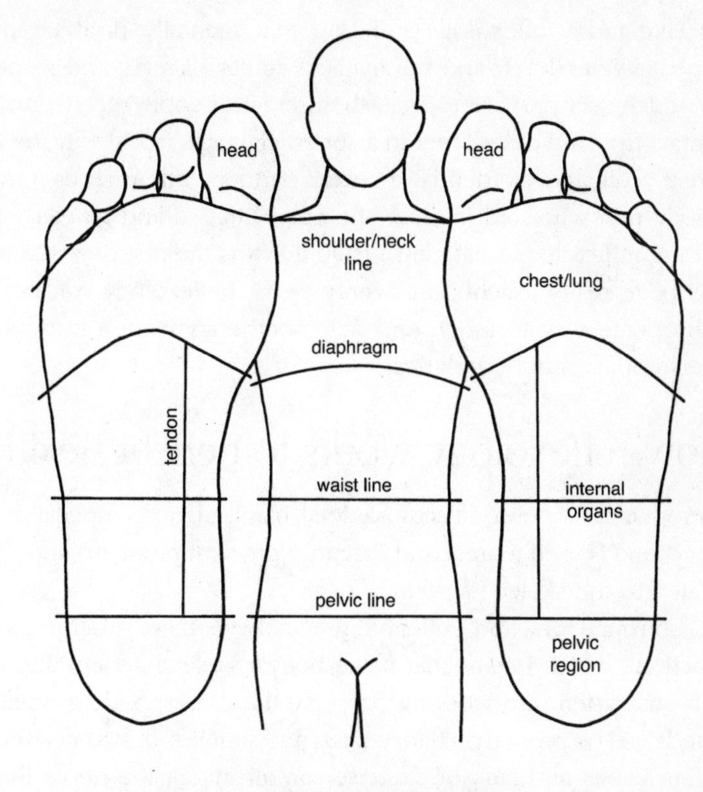

The foot is divided into cross-sections

firm, so that the feet feel secure, but there should not be so much pressure that it causes discomfort.

Reflexologists use the sensitivity of the foot to tune into the body and stimulate its various parts by pressing a tiny reflex and sending a vital force to the part that needs help. There are hundreds of these minute reflexes, and a sensitive touch and pressure can locate a reflex that may correspond to the corner of the eye or a particular portion of the small intestine.

Touch

Even before you start treating someone with reflexology, touch is a wonderful healing gift in itself. First greet the feet by holding them firmly and using the basic relaxation techniques described on p. 82 – relaxing the feet relaxes the entire body.

Like most reflexologists, I find that mentally disabled people, hyperactive children and traumatised adults all relax and respond to my touch as I prepare to treat them. Some people receive no tactile contact from anyone except in a superficial or practical way, be it from carers, colleagues, friends or even partners. In America I met an elderly nun who told me that she often hugged and greeted visitors, but the reflexology treatment I gave her was the first time she felt she had been really touched in twenty years. Reflexology can be a very appropriate way to touch and help soothe someone's body without overstepping any boundaries.

How reflexology works to benefit health

Chiropractic is neuromusculoskeletal manipulation, especially of the spine, and is used to treat and diagnose physical problems and diseases related to the skeletal system.

Chiropractors and reflexologists believe that 'structure governs function', which means that if the body's skeletal system and central nervous system are working properly the corresponding organs and glands will be properly balanced, fed and stimulated. Bad posture, poor eating habits and lack of exercise can all impair the nerve functions of the body, with drastic results. Reflexology works precisely on the skeletal and nervous systems, to help the body adjust. It has been said that reflexology reaches the parts that other therapies cannot reach. It certainly allows the body to relax to a state of calm normally experienced after meditation or a good night's sleep. One of reflexology's great contributions to general well-being is that it improves the circulation, stimulates the lymphatic system and helps to cleanse the body of toxins.

Case study

After I had treated a young girl with VRT for her lower back problems she reported that her irritable bowel had become much more stable in the process. She had not even told me about this problem, but I had worked the lower back reflexes and one of the nerves from the lumbar vertebrae is connected to the colon. The body had simply experienced release in the spine, and the knock-on effect was a calmer bowel.

Fight, flight and stress

When treating other people, impress upon them that the reflexes are energetic and a slight tenderness is a sign of vitality – a good thing, and not something to worry about. So try not to fall into the trap of identifying tender spots, such as the liver or the uterus, as you work.

Almost everyone's adrenal reflexes are tender, as we need a certain level of the hormone adrenalin to keep us active and alert. We need our adrenalin working when we run for the bus or slam on the car brakes to avoid an accident. This is the 'fight or flight' mechanism that is essential to the survival of all living creatures. But while it is indispensable when we need to fight off danger or run from it, if we live at that high level of tension all the time – as we sit in traffic jams on the way to work, or cope with screaming children and aged parents, or try to deal with a demanding boss and unsupportive colleagues – it can be very destructive. High adrenalin levels can also be positive for a short while when we are enjoying ourselves.

> **No more crying babies!**
>
> Small babies respond wonderfully to gentle strokes on their reflexes, and family doctors often send me parents with tiny colicky infants. I treat the child synergistically, using hand and foot reflexes, and then teach the parents a few simple techniques to calm the digestive system. When a stranger came up to me in a Bristol supermarket and thanked me for giving him a good night's sleep I was somewhat startled. Then he told me that his wife had just pointed me out as the 'foot lady' who had stopped their offspring from screaming half the night!

Over 70 per cent of disease is stress-related – not only obvious conditions such as irritable bowel and stomach ulcers, but also other problems ranging from stiff necks and headaches to chronic illness. Reflexology, as already explained, helps the body to unwind, relax and then heal itself. Conversely, if you feel very lethargic and tired you should work the same adrenal reflexes to get the opposite effect. How can this be achieved? Because reflexology is concerned with allowing our systems to achieve a natural balance and, if there is insufficient adrenalin circulating, the body can be stimulated via reflexology to secrete more of the hormone. If we are overstressed, the calming pressure of our fingertips on the reflexes will help the body to lower our adrenalin levels.

The same balancing technique works when you are treating high or low blood pressure. The heart, diaphragm, spinal and endocrine (hormonal) reflexes are worked for both conditions, and then the body itself is allowed to get on with the actual healing mechanisms.

Reflexology and the system of zones

All reflexologists study the system of the ten longitudinal zones in the body, five per foot, that divide the body into segments (see diagram below). These are the conduits for the flow of energy from the foot and hand reflexes to the corresponding parts of the body. It is helpful to visualise these three-dimensional zones as ten slices of the body in equal proportion, with zone one running from the big toes and thumb and ending with zone five, which runs from the little fingers and toes.

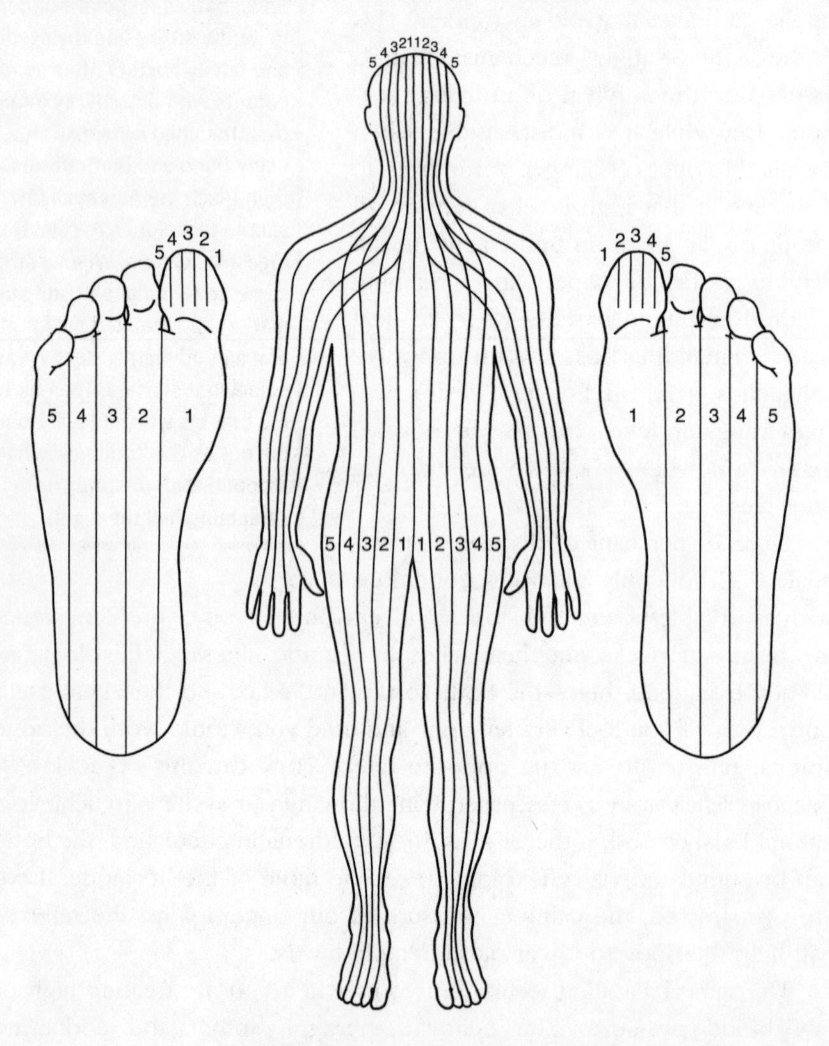

The ten longitudinal energy zones of the body

It was Dr Fitzgerald, early in the twentieth century, who suggested that energy flowed through these zones from the toes to the head. It followed that the energy could be blocked at any point by dis-ease in the body. This in turn can weaken other organs and glands within the same zone. For example, the kidney and eye are both in the third zone, and I have had several clients who have complained of problems in both body parts.

In recent decades the zones have tended to take second place to the reflexes on the sole as the focus of interest. Yet the new type of reflexology, Vertical Reflex Therapy, appears to activate the zones in an unprecedented way. There seems to be a faster and more direct line of communication between the reflexes and the parts of the body when the feet are weight-bearing. Not only that, but congestion in another part of the body can be very quickly over-ridden. Many people report a rush of warmth or energy as they experience VRT, followed by clicks, twinges and twitches as the body makes numerous adjustments to regain its balance fast.

I believe that the zones themselves can become congested and that VRT manages to recharge and clear these energy lines, thus accelerating the healing processes. The Zonal Triggers described in Chapter 7 are ankle reflexes that play an important role in activating the zones at great speed so that the body is more receptive to healing.

VRT brings a new dimension

When a person is standing for a VRT treatment it is the top (dorsum) of the foot which is worked and not, as in conventional reflexology, the sole (plantar). In *Reflexology – Art, Science and History* Christine Issel illustrates many interesting and ancient charts of the feet from cultures around the world. They do not correspond precisely to the charts that modern reflexologists use, which shows that reflexology is an inexact science that will always be open to new ideas and interpretations.

Why does VRT achieve even better results?

Like many others, I am intrigued to know exactly why VRT is proving to be so effective. My theory is that the upright body appears to be in a position of increased vitality because it is weight-bearing: the muscles are taut, there is pressure on the bones to support the upright skeleton, and the heart is pumping oxygenated blood to the organs, which, in a standing position, will be less impacted by possible bad posture.

In addition, although the standing foot reflexes have a more vital response, I suggest that VRT puts the body into *neutral* – a state in which the long-term legacy of strain, tension, degeneration and scar tissue in an organ or muscle is bypassed to allow direct access to the original problem. This would explain why, at many VRT workshops, whiplash injuries, chronic stomach pain and stiff knees and hips have dramatically improved, often within minutes of treatment.

What you need to know about basic reflexology before giving a VRT treatment

Trained reflexologists will have no problem assimilating all the new information on VRT, because they will be building on an existing knowledge of the reflexes, anatomy and physiology, together with some advanced reflexology techniques they will have learnt as their career has developed. Although I use my knuckles and lubricating cream, as Anthony Porter teaches his students, it is not essential to use these methods. The necessary finger and thumb movements can be administered in the familiar ways that the therapist has already learnt.

Readers who are new to reflexology will find in this book all the information they need to enable them to practise VRT and the associated techniques. With basic VRT, it is possible to bring about excellent results even if you are not a reflexologist. If you do want to become a reflexologist, there are some good introductory books on the subject and some excellent training courses (see p. 183).

And now why not experience a first taste of VRT with this short treatment? I call it the VRT Revitaliser.

'Is it all right for a non-professional to give VRT and conventional reflexology to family and friends?'

VRT can help people with a huge number of common conditions (see Chapter 10). As an amateur you can safely give a powerful Basic VRT treatment by following the guidelines in Chapter 5, but avoid treating women who are under four months pregnant, and people with deep vein thrombosis, epilepsy, heart problems, infectious skin diseases, and varicose veins. Cancer and ME are two conditions that respond well to VRT – carers can be taught by professional reflexologists to give gentle, specific VRT treatments.

VRT Revitaliser – a five-minute treatment

This is a simple way to release stress and loosen a stiff back or neck, especially after sitting or driving for a long time. The final pinch of the big toes is very energising.

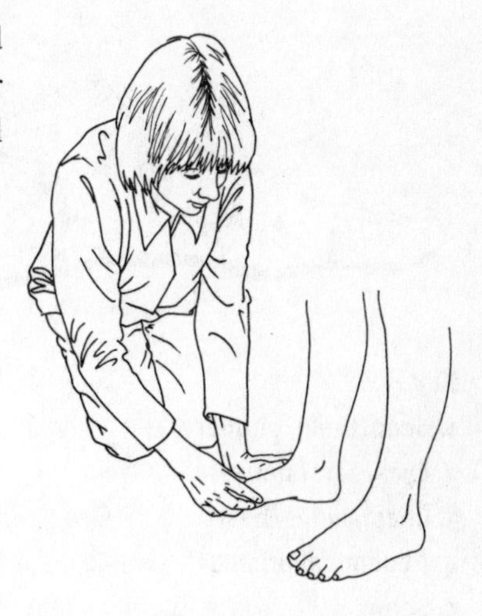

Requirements:

- Two people – one acts as client and the other as the therapist. The roles can then be reversed.
- A towel or mat on which to stand.
- A cushion to kneel on.
- A table or chair nearby for support in case the person being treated becomes unsteady.
- Space to move around the person being treated.

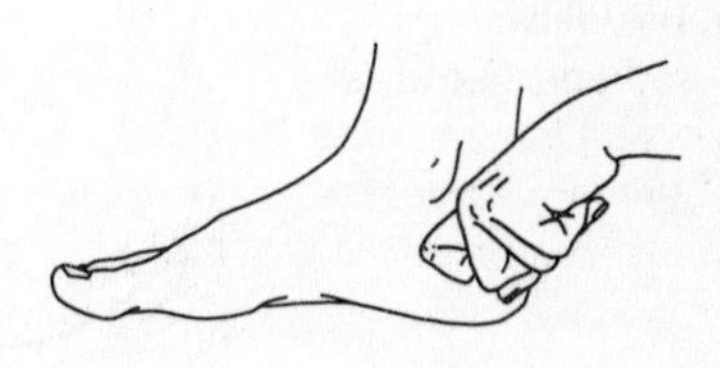

1. The 'client' stands on a mat with bare feet, slightly apart, facing the 'therapist'.
2. The therapist sits or kneels and, placing both hands on the client's right foot, uses their fingertips, or knuckles, to press and gently massage the flesh around the client's ankles, using a rotating movement. Use a tiny amount of a non-oily cream, if you like, to help lubricate your fingertips. Working on the ankles like this helps to stimulate hip/pelvic/sciatic reflexes and the reproductive system. Now stroke across the top of the right ankle, making brushing movements with your thumbs. This helps boost the immune system. Repeat from the beginning for the left foot.

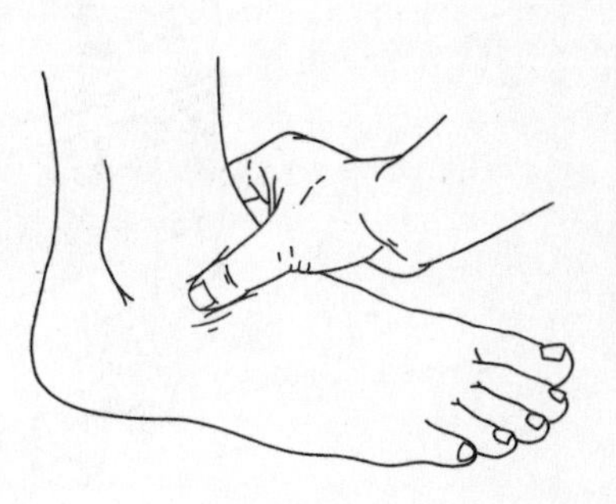

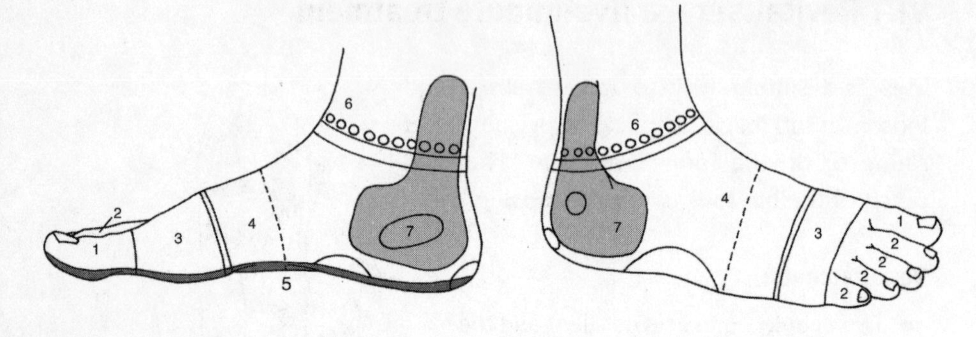

Key

1. Head/brain/pituitary

2. Eyes/ears/sinuses

3. Chest/lungs/heart

4. Abdominal organs

5. Spine

6. Groin/helper heart and diaphram/Zonal Triggers

7. Hip/pelvic/reproductive area

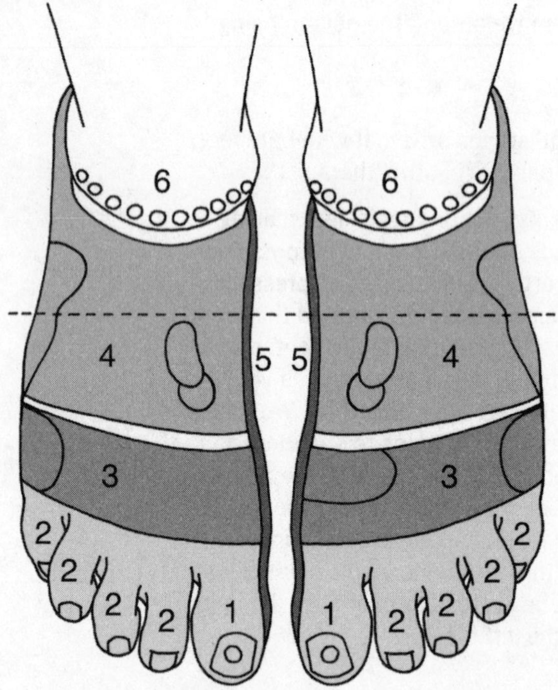

A simplified VRT foot chart

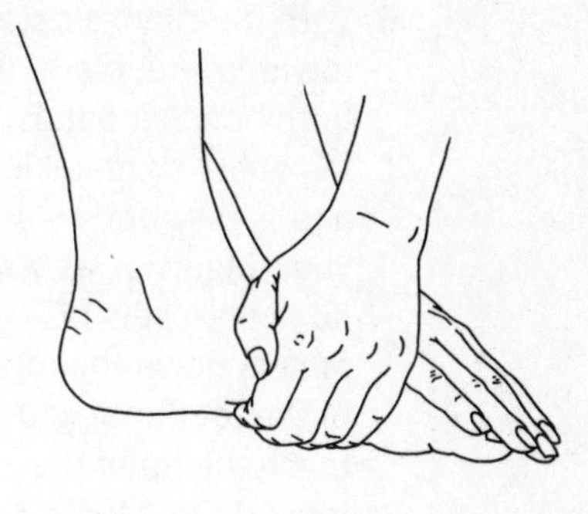

3. The next three moves are made first on the right foot and then, after the client has turned to face the other way, on the left foot:

   - Ask the client to turn sideways so that he or she is facing your right. Press your left palm firmly on the top of the client's foot to steady it.
   - With your right hand, tuck your fingers under the client's right instep and pull gently upwards as if stretching the instep. Do not move your fingers – let them act as a handle to ease the instep a fraction. This helps stimulate the lower back reflexes.

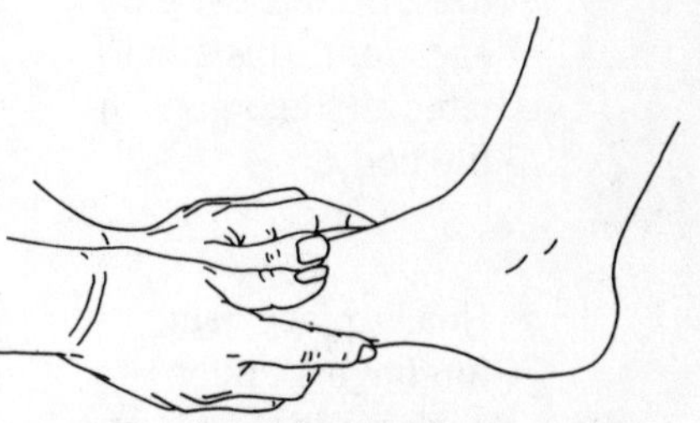

   - Press your forefinger up and down the inside edge of the foot, following its natural arch, from the side of the big toenail to the ankle/heel area. This, too, stimulates the reflexes in the back.

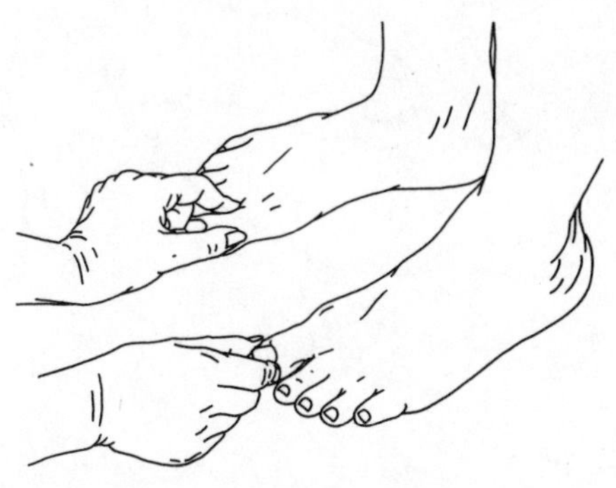

4. With the client facing you, using one hand on each foot, simultaneously pinch down the sides of each toe and rotate your fingers on the top of each toe. Work outwards from the big toes.

5. Return to the big toes and gently rotate your fingertips at the base of each toe simultaneously. Work outwards from the big toe. This helps the sinuses, ears, eyes, chest and immune system.

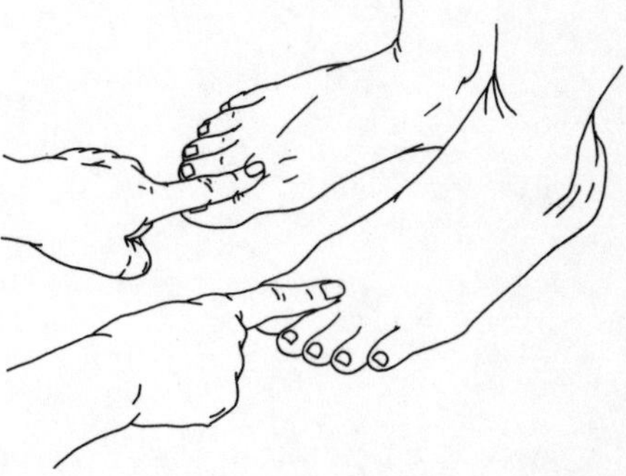

6. With the client's back towards you, place both hands around his or her right ankle and press gently with your fingertips as you edge both sets of fingers down the top of the foot until you reach the tip of the toes. Do this twice on each foot. This stimulates all the organs in the body.

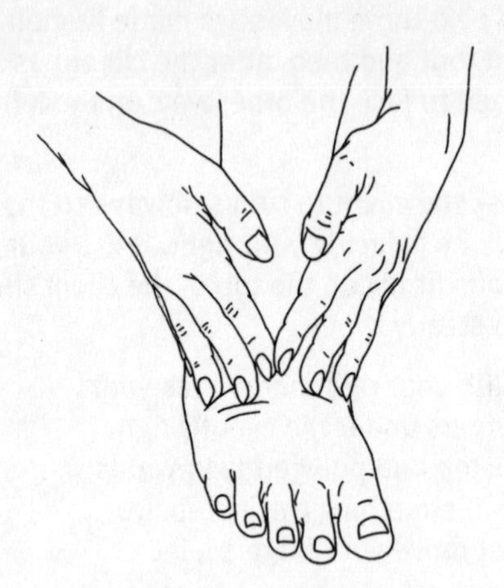

7. Finally, place your forefingers under each big toe, nails on the ground. Rest your thumbs on top of the toenail and pinch the toes as the client leans very slightly forward to increase the pressure. This energising movement, which helps balance the hormonal reflexes, completes the treatment.

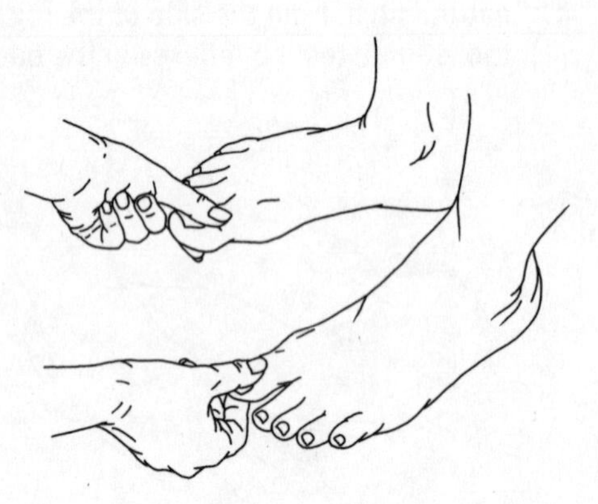

Key differences between VRT and conventional reflexology

Terms not yet explained, such as Synergistic Reflexology, Zonal Triggers and Diaphragm Rocking, will be fully covered later.

- VRT is practised on the feet/hands in a standing, weight-bearing position. Conventional reflexology is practised on the feet/hands in a reclining position.
- Synergistic Reflexology (see Chapter 6) applies to the simultaneous working of specific hand and foot reflexes.
- VRT self-help techniques (see Chapter 9) enable you to self-treat much more sensitively and effectively than is possible with conventional reflexology, using hands and feet in standing and seated positions.
- Most VRT techniques can be used during conventional reflexology sessions as well.
- A fully comprehensive Complete VRT treatment (see Chapter 7) lasts twenty minutes. Most reflexology treatments are between thirty and sixty minutes.
- The body responds very quickly to VRT, sometimes instantaneously in orthopaedic conditions.
- VRT approaches the plantar (sole of the foot) reflexes via the dorsal area (on top of the foot).
- New and deeper reflexes for use with VRT have been located on the feet and hands.
- VRT identifies specific new ankle reflexes called Zonal Triggers that, when combined with two specific hand and foot reflexes, help to accelerate the natural healing process.
- Diaphragm Rocking (see Chapters 6 and 7), a technique used to consolidate VRT, appears to prioritise the body's weaknesses and pumps energy to the parts most in need of stimulation or healing.

The systems of the body and their functions

WE NATURALLY ASSUME ALL IS WELL IN OUR BODY UNTIL IT TELLS US OTHERWISE. We never think about what our knee, nose or stomach is doing, for example, until something goes wrong and we are made aware of it through pain or discomfort. And yet our bodies are dealing with thousands of different functions and making checks, compensations and balances every second of the day. The delicate balance between good health and illness is very fragile, and yet the miracle of life is that the body continues to repair, support and compensate for accidents, poor diet and the general wear and tear of ageing.

The systems of the body comprise groups of organs, glands, nerves and skeletal structures, each of which performs a specific function. The function of the digestive system, for example, is to process food and drink, to extract the necessary nutrients from what is consumed and disperse them through the body, and then excrete the surplus as waste matter. The endocrine system controls our hormonal function; many women know how a tiny imbalance in their hormones can create premenstrual or menopausal symptoms. Men, too, undergo hormonal changes as they age, which can result in loss of libido or impotence.

This chapter briefly describes the systems of the body and talks about the reflexes relevant to Vertical Reflex Therapy techniques. The systems of the body are:

The neurological system

The entire body is controlled by the brain and the central nervous system. The spinal cord supplies nerves and relays messages to and from the appropriate parts of the body to the brain.

The skeletal system

This consists of the bones that protect and support the body.

The muscular system

There are three different types of muscle that support the skeletal system, giving strength to the body and enabling it to move.

The lymphatic system

This deals with disposing of waste in the body by means of lymph nodes, tissues and vessels.

The respiratory system

This takes in oxygen via the lungs to nourish the blood, and discharges carbon dioxide also via the lungs.

The cardiovascular and circulatory system

This includes the heart and the blood, which circulates through the veins, arteries and capillaries.

The digestive system

This processes food into chemical substances to nourish the body, and excretes the waste products.

The urinary system

This processes toxins from the blood via the kidneys, which not only act as a filter for urine but controls the balance of many chemical functions in the body.

The endocrine system

This consists of ductless glands that produce hormones to stimulate and control many of the body's processes, including metabolism.

The sense organs

These include the skin, ears, nose, tongue and eyes, all of which give the brain information about the body's environment.

The reproductive system

This consists of a series of organs which among other things produce sperm (male) and eggs or ova (female) from the ovaries to produce a baby.

The value of a holistic therapy

Reflexology's holistic approach comes into its own when treating the systems of the body through the feet, because they are all worked systematically. VRT, and indeed all reflexology treatments, always treat every part of the body through the feet and then return to the areas that felt tender or relate to a known weakness in the body. The energetic pathways are stimulated enabling the malfunctioning parts to respond, which in turn allows the body to function better.

If I work the pituitary gland reflex on the big toe, which is the master gland or control for the endocrine system, I am trying to help balance the entire hormonal system. I will then work the adrenal, thyroid and other glands in anticipation that the knock-on effect will be healthier hormones. A month later a client may report that she has had a less painful period, or a man might say that his libido has increased. In both cases I will have worked the ovary/testes reflex, but I may not know, and do not even need to know, which particular reflex I worked to help achieve that result. I just worked the correct reflexes connected with the endocrine system as described in this chapter and let the body get on with balancing any irregularities.

The tenderness or improvement in the feel of a certain reflex may give an indication of which endocrine gland was imbalanced. Reflexologists receive confirmation of this when a client has blood tests which show, for example, that the thyroid gland is under functioning and the thyroid reflex on the base of the big toe is the only tender endocrine reflex.

With VRT the reflexes become extremely sensitive, which is an extra helpful indicator of where there is an imbalance in the body. (Some clients might even complain that reflexology was a pleasant experience until they experienced VRT – though they would be the first to admit that a couple of painful jabs to the feet while standing is a small price to pay for instant relief in some cases.) Someone may complain of shoulder pain but it is the neck and lumbar spinal reflexes that prove to be painful, so I will be guided by that information and concentrate on those areas. In other words I will focus on other parts of the skeletal system, using as my guide the feel of the reflexes and feedback from the client regarding sensitivity. I will, of course, work the shoulder as well to consolidate my work.

Reflexologists are able to concentrate on particular areas of weakness but, as already explained, they are not treating specific diseases or diagnosing what is wrong, as a medical practitioner would. Chapter 10 contains instructions for treating certain conditions from sinus problems to backache, but, while it is true that you can focus on a specific problem or illness, at the end of the day it is the body that will try to make the appropriate changes and adjustments. An informed approach to the workings of the body and the reflexes on the foot is all you need in order to help someone. So, while it is essential to have a general overview of how the body's systems work, it is not necessary to try to remember all the details below.

Qualified reflexologists, who are already trained in anatomy and physiology, can bypass most of this chapter. They will appreciate the new VRT techniques which will help them as they use their skills to fine-tune the body's various systems.

'Can VRT be used as a preventative treatment?'

Yes, because the body is stimulated to heal itself and maintain its health. This applies whether you are young or old, an athlete or a sedentary office worker.

Understanding the body's functions – beauty is more than skin-deep

The human body is a complex sum of many parts, and all its systems rely on each other to maintain a healthy balance and function properly. Reflexology's main aim of bringing about balance is achieved by stimulating all these systems so that they function better and more effectively. Some people's diet, for instance, comprises mainly fast foods, sweets and carbonated sugary drinks with little fresh fruit and vegetables. After a while their skin may become spotty or they may begin to suffer from indigestion. The advertising message is to buy a particular brand of blemish cream or antacid pill to cure the problem. These people may be much happier with the superficial approach of treating the symptoms and not the cause, because to look deeper into what is going on inside the body is more threatening. The body will go on adjusting and adapting for a long time as it accommodates our bad posture, lack of exercise and unhealthy eating habits. But no part of the body works in isolation from the rest and we owe it to ourselves to look after our bodies.

Looking after your health

Good health is one of our most precious possessions, and one of the easiest ways in which we can help ourselves is to become aware of our body's needs. The important points to remember are:

- exercise
- nutrition
- sleep
- fluids.

Gyms and sports centres are now very popular and often oversubscribed, but it is always best to find out what is right for you as an individual. Why pace on a treadmill in a gym if you would rather be running across the park? Set yourself small, realistic goals and achieve them, rather than formulating a rigorous plan more suited to a professional athlete. It also sometimes helps to share your exercise regime with a friend or family member. This makes for good discipline too, because mutual support will help you both to keep up the commitment.

As far as nutrition is concerned, most people are now aware that they should be eating more fruit and vegetables and less fat. But do seek proper dietary advice before radically changing your eating habits. And don't go overboard with supplements – many people I treat have a cupboard full of half-empty bottles of vitamin pills which they bought ages ago, and can't even remember why they wanted them in the first place. Professional nutritional advice can be invaluable but if you do decide to take a supplement, be aware that many of the more expensive brands are better value than their cheaper counterparts, because they tend to contain more effective quantities of the key ingredients and are better quality.

Sleep is the most healing time of all for both our bodies and our minds. A decent night's sleep is, ideally, eight hours, but seven is sufficient for most people. If you have trouble sleeping, try some of the natural herbal or homeopathic remedies now available in chemists as well as health food shops.

Finally, drink more water – lots more! Six to eight glasses a day will make a world of difference to the way your body functions. The human body consists of 75 per cent water, and all our organs and

Case study

A cautionary tale: A youngish business man came to me suffering from irritable bowel, haemorrhoids (piles) and flatulence. He always felt worse after his canteen lunch each day or following a rich evening meal. I asked him to keep a brief diary of what he had eaten prior to a bad attack of digestive trouble.

He improved a little with VRT and reflexology, but found that rich dairy products, sugar and pork would give him diarrhoea and stomach pains. I taught him how to work the stomach reflex on his left hand after a meal to help him to produce enough digestive enzymes. His haemorrhoids shrunk very quickly with VRT but he was most unwilling to give up his favourite foods as he maintained that 'a little of what you fancy does you good'! This was despite the fact I repeatedly told him that a little of what *irritated* his system did him a lot of harm.

He continued to eat what he liked as he felt that VRT kept the symptoms at bay without him having to take control of his own eating habits. This state of affairs continued until he moved away and ceased his reflexology treatments. I recently heard that he was suffering from an inflammation of the bowel and was awaiting hospital tests. This is an example of a condition that improved with VRT and illustrates the consequences of failing to read our bodies' messages.

muscles respond better when properly hydrated. Remember that thirst is not the brain's first sign of dehydration, but the last, so always keep up your fluid intake. If water (the purest form of fluid) is not available, substitute weak tea, herbal teas, soft drinks or fruit juice, but bear in mind that some of these contain sugar, stimulants and other substances, the intake of which is best kept to a minimum. Enjoy a moderate intake of alcohol, as it has a dehydrating effect on the body. Coffee should be avoided if possible. In other words, water is best – read Dr F. Batmanghelidj's book *Your Body's Many Cries for Water* to understand why water is the elixir of life.

The neurological system

The neurological system consists of the central nervous system and the autonomic nervous system.

The central nervous system

The CNS or central nervous system supplies information to the body via twelve pairs of cranial nerves at the base of the brain and thirty-one pairs of spinal nerves that branch out down the length of the spinal cord to every part of the body. The CNS is highly complex and reflexologists treat it by simplified guidelines

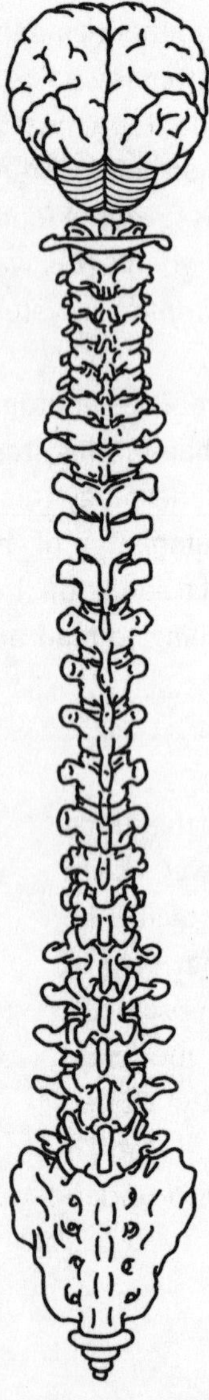

The brain and spinal cord encased by vertebrae

The twelve cranial nerves stem from the base of the brain and supply functions within the head, including the operation of the eyes, the sense of smell and the facial muscles.

The thirty-one pairs of spinal nerves

These comprise:

- Eight pairs of cervical nerves, from seven vertebrae, which emanate from the neck and supply the lips, sinuses and throat among others.
- Twelve pairs of thoracic nerves situated in the upper thoracic spine, which serve the lungs, adrenal glands and kidneys among other organs.
- Five pairs of lumbar nerves which stem from the vertebrae of the lower back and are linked to parts of the body in the pelvic region and legs such as the reproductive organs, the bladder, and the feet and ankles.
- Sacral and coccyx nerves, which consist of five sacral nerves, also serving the bladder, plus hips, buttocks and the coccygeal nerve which is linked to the rectum and anus.

How reflexology and VRT help

It is not necessary to remember the names of these nerves and their functions unless you are a professional reflexologist. In Chapter 8, on advanced VRT techniques, the nerve reflexes will be linked to the organ reflexes. Here your overall knowledge of how the body works, plus access to the chart of the central nervous system, will enable you to link the points of the neural pathway reflex with a part of the body that is unbalanced. For example, a tender uterus reflex on the foot (below the inside ankle) can be linked to the spinal nerve reflex (L3) on the inner edge of the foot that may well also be tender, and the two points are then worked together. Working the specific nerve reflex and the corresponding organ or gland at the same time has produced exceptional results for VRT practitioners.

The spinal nerves supply messages to every part of the body, and if the spinal vertebrae which protect the spinal cord are compressed or damaged then the corresponding organ can also be affected. A heavy fall on the coccyx at the base of the spine can cause a vertebra to become very slightly misaligned and this could result, for example, in temporary, or even permanent, bladder problems if the nerve is damaged or trapped. Most references to trapped nerves are associated with back pain, and it is much more effective to have an osteopathic treatment or massage to help release the nerve than to resort to painkillers, which only mask the problem. Vertical Reflex Therapy is now a powerful new option to help release trapped nerves.

The autonomic nervous system

The ANS or autonomic nervous system controls all the body's systems over which we have no voluntary control. It has two parts – the sympathetic system and the parasympathetic system.

The sympathetic nervous system has several functions including increasing the heart rate, mobilising glucose and stimulating the sweat glands. It is involved in helping the body cope with increased activity.

The parasympathetic nervous system helps to lower blood pressure and reduce the pace of the heartbeat, and is involved more with the functions of the body when at rest.

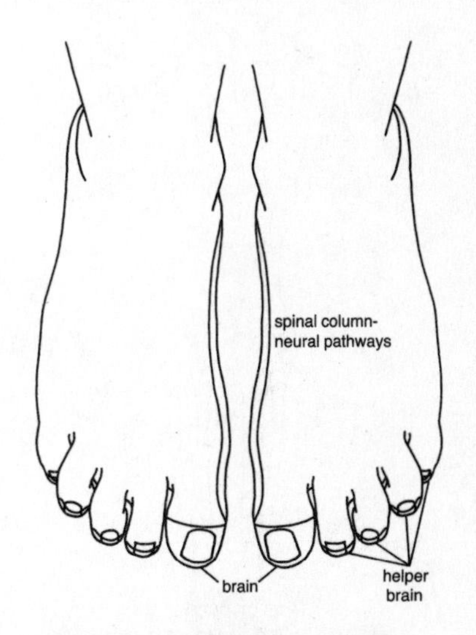

Position of neurological reflexes on the feet

How reflexology and VRT help

VRT and reflexology in general work on the autonomic nervous system in an indirect way by treating the whole body through the feet and triggering a response where needed. I have treated many people with high blood pressure, and over a period of time their doctors have often been able to reduce their medication because the body is regulating the blood pressure itself. I did not work on a specific point but simply treated the reflexes of the heart, diaphragm and associated helper areas for the heart. In doing so the parasympathetic nervous system was able to respond naturally and work better to regulate the blood pressure.

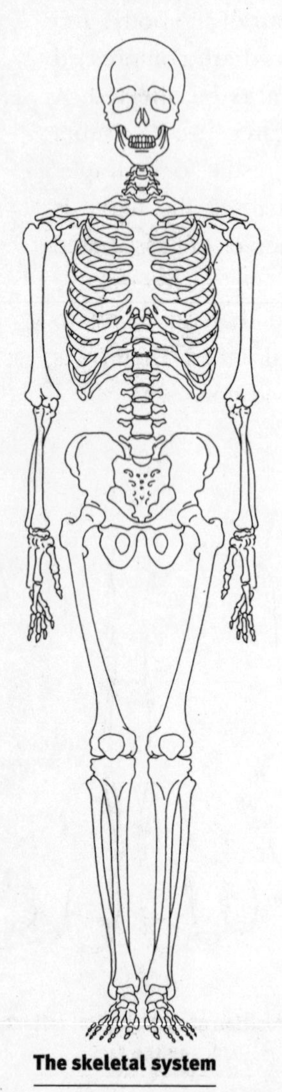

The skeletal system

The skeletal system

The skeletal system has two main functions, protection and movement, and is the principal support of the body. It contains 206 bones – twenty-six of them are in each foot and twenty-seven in each hand! The bones are made of dense tissue but are very much alive and active, consisting of 45 per cent minerals, 30 per cent organic material and 25 per cent water.

The bones that protect the body are:

- the skull, which protects the brain
- the ribcage, which protects the heart and lungs
- the spinal column, which protects the spinal cord
- the pelvic bones, which offer some protection to abdominal organs.

The second function of the skeleton is to provide movement to the body. The bones undertake numerous chemical activities and produce and store minerals. The individual bones attach to the tendons and muscles and assist in the formation of red blood cells and some white blood cells in the bone marrow. The skull and brain are extremely heavy, and yet are comfortably supported on the narrow cervical vertebrae in the neck. Looking at a skeleton, it is obvious what an impact it has on the nerve supply and circulation of the blood. Pressure on the organs can result if the spine is out of alignment – a flexible, upright spine is the key to good health and vitality.

How reflexology and VRT help

VRT practitioners and some reflexologists use the bones of the hands and feet as pointers to chart the exact position of the reflexes. The navicular bones, for example, on the feet mark the waistline of the human body when related to the mapping out of the feet.

VRT has been particularly successful in loosening up the joints in the body and helping skeletal and mobility problems. Synergistic VRT (see p. 105), where the hand and foot are worked simultaneously, appears to free up tight muscles and allows limbs to revert to their correct position naturally.

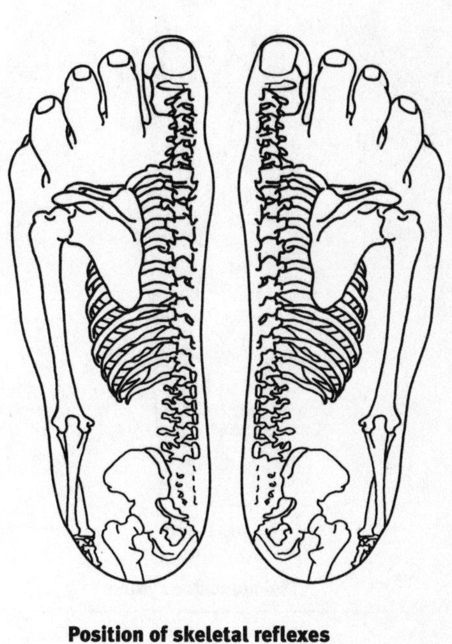

Position of skeletal reflexes on the feet

The muscular system

Designed to allow us to move, the muscular system is responsible for about 50 per cent of our body weight. It is made up of two types of muscles, voluntary and involuntary.

Voluntary muscles

These are used for movement such as running or raising an arm, and are under our conscious control. They make up about 25 per cent of our body weight, and are striped or cross-banded.

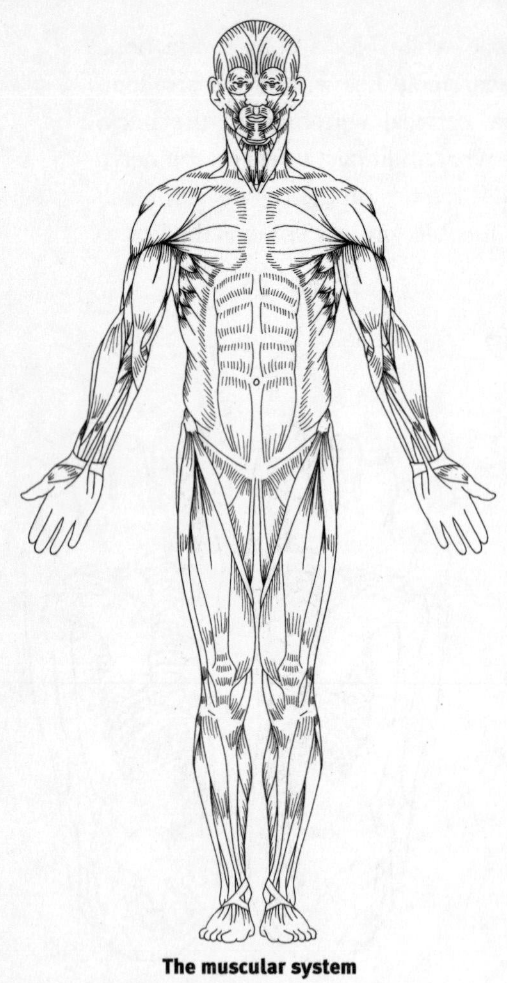

The muscular system

Involuntary muscles

These are not under direct conscious control. The heart and digestive system, for instance, use muscles that are not consciously controlled by the brain. These muscles are called smooth muscles.

All voluntary muscles have two points of attachment to the bones. The origin is the anchor, and does not move; the insertion applies to the bone of attachment, where it does move.

Gentle regular exercise can tone up the muscles and enable them to retain their elasticity. Often muscles will go into spasm, resulting in pain and decreased mobility. This can happen due to overuse or underuse, and the feeling of stiffness is the result of the presence of too many waste products in the system which stops the muscular fibres sliding over each other easily.

Tendons

These are dense cords of connective tissue that connect the centre of the muscle to the bone. They have no elasticity, only strength; reflexologists work gently on the tendon and do not apply pressure. On the foot, the tendon is located on the medial sole and is situated parallel to the instep. In VRT, of course, this aspect is usually irrelevant because the sole is not touched except in two advanced techniques.

Ligaments

These are connective tissues that hold bone to bone, and have some elasticity – enough to prevent the bones from dislocating and permit slight freedom of movement.

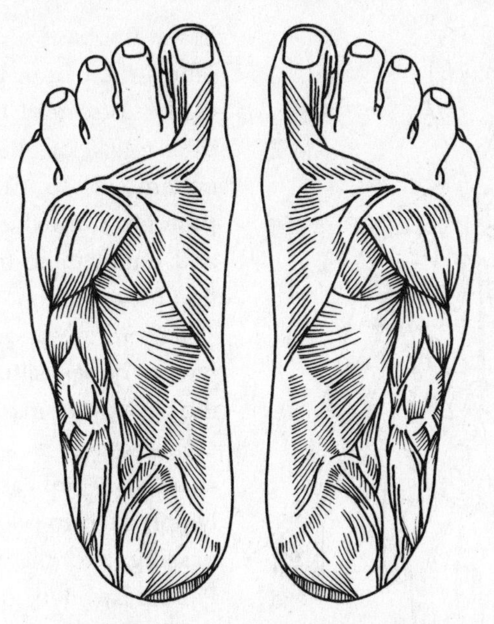

Position of muscular reflexes on the feet

How reflexology and VRT help

VRT has had remarkable success in freeing up tense muscles instantaneously. Shoulders and necks respond particularly well, as do hip joints. Many people who have had hip replacements have experienced relief from soreness and irritation of the surrounding muscles after receiving VRT.

The lymphatic system

This system comprises lymph vessels and lymph nodes. The lymphatic system is crucial to the health of the body as its role is to carry waste matter, excess fluid and toxins from the cells and tissues. The white blood cells in the body are known as lymphocytes, and it is essential for the body to maintain the correct white blood cell count in its fight against disease. The tonsils, adenoids, spleen and thymus gland are also part of the lymphatic system.

There are two main drainage points in the body for lymph: the thoracic duct and the right lymphatic duct. The thoracic duct drains waste products from the legs, pelvic and abdominal area and the left half of the upper body, including the head. The right lymphatic duct

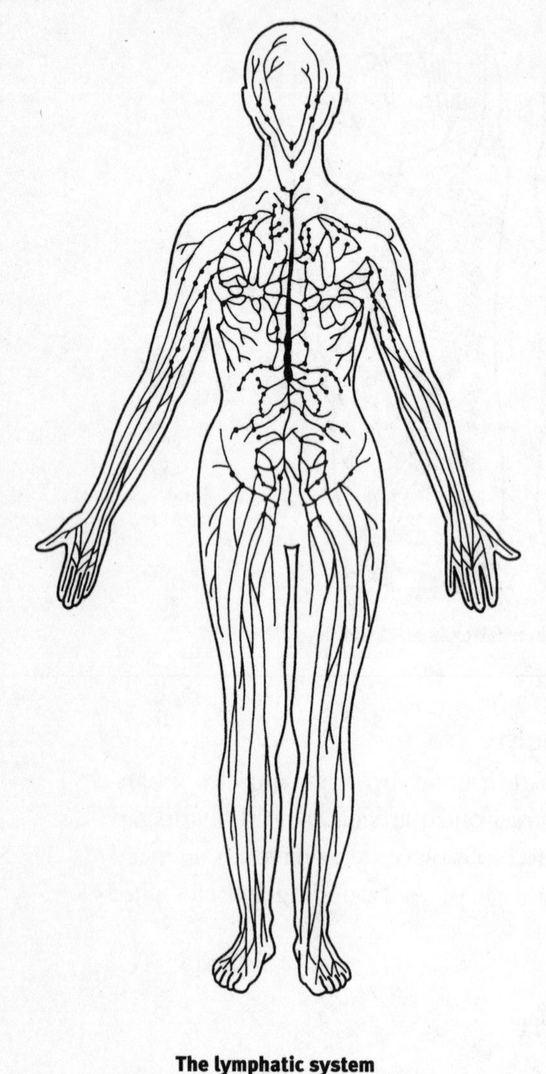
The lymphatic system

lies at the base of the neck and drains fluid from the right side of the torso and head. One of the roles of the lymphatic system is to remove large proteins from the body tissue and return them to the circulation for excretion.

There are about a hundred lymph nodes situated all over the body, with many in the neck area. As large as a peanut or as small as a pinhead, they act as lymph filters to prevent infection passing into the bloodstream. Painful swollen glands are the result of the lymph nodes being overwhelmed by toxins due to illness or infection in the body: they swell because they cannot process the waste products quickly enough.

The lymph system also has a vital role to play in supporting the immune system. A healthy lymph system means a healthy body, as disease and bacteria are efficiently eliminated.

Tissue fluid

This is colourless and is derived from blood plasma. Tissue fluid seeps through the capillaries (the smallest blood vessels) but, unlike blood, it is not pumped from the heart. Instead it is moved by exercise and taking deep breaths. When the tissue fluid reaches the lymph vessels it is called lymph. One of the best ways of helping lymph to circulate through your body is to use a Rebounder which is a small trampoline that is used for five to ten minutes daily. The lymph system can become very sluggish due to lack of exercise and apparently as much lymph flows in ten minutes of bouncing as it does during a forty minute run. Rebounders are one metre in diameter with 20cm screw-on feet for flat storage, they cost about £70 and can be obtained from John Lewis stores and sports shops.

The tonsils and adenoids

These are part of the lymph system and are situated at the back of the nasal cavity.

The spleen

This consists of lymphoid tissue and is a major filter system for damaged cells. It also stores iron and breaks down old red blood cells.

The thymus

This gland plays an important role in the immune system of children and shrinks at puberty. Its function is hormonal, stimulating the body to produce lymphocytes and lymph tissue. The role of the thymus in adults is being reviewed, as there is a suggestion that it is still functioning and involved in the production of cells called T-lymphocytes which are vital in the body's fight against tumour-producing cells.

How reflexology and VRT help

Reflexology has always achieved impressive results when it comes to lymph drainage and related conditions such as oedema in the feet. With VRT the standing position can accelerate the movement of fluid through the body, so a reduction of fluid and a healthier lymphatic system may well be noticeable immediately. Often the improvements in lymph drainage are more permanent or only require a monthly VRT treatment to keep the problem at bay.

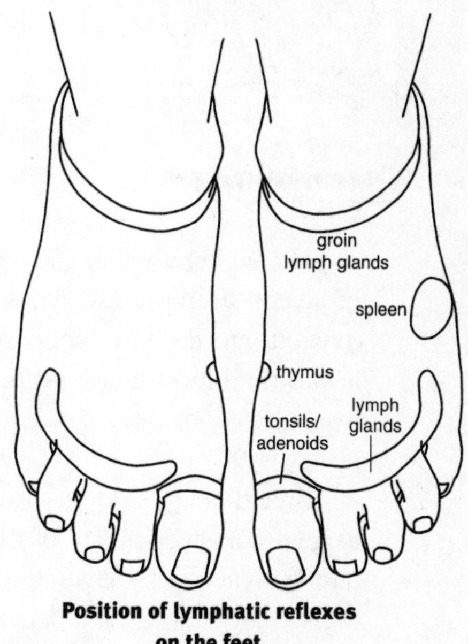

Position of lymphatic reflexes on the feet

The respiratory system

The respiratory system's organs are basically related to breathing in oxygen (inspiration) and exhaling carbon dioxide and some water (expiration). The purpose of breathing is to oxygenate the blood, upon which every cell depends. The system is divided into the upper and lower respiratory tracts.

Upper respiratory tract organs

These include the mouth, throat, larynx, cilia (filters) and the sinus cavities in the head. As air passes through the nose it is filtered and warmed before passing into the lungs.

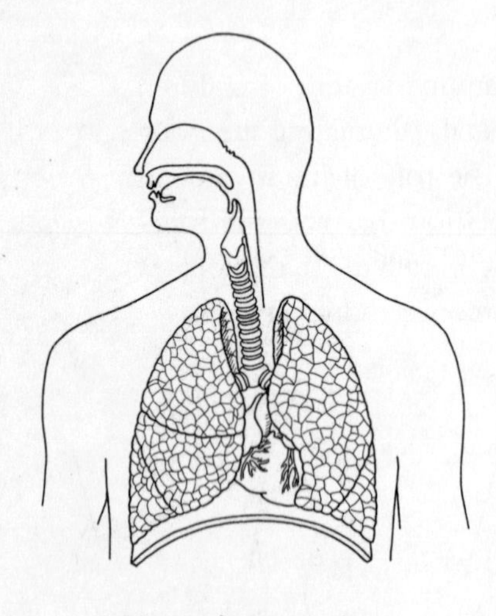

The respiratory system

Lower respiratory tract organs

These include the windpipe (trachea), the bronchi and the lungs. The lungs themselves comprise the alveoli (air sacs), bronchioles and bronchial tubes.

The lungs are the main organ of the respiratory tract, and the diaphragm is a large muscular wall that points upwards towards the lungs. When the diaphragm contracts, during inspiration, the atmospheric pressure on the lungs decreases, causing the air to rush in. When the opposite happens and the diaphragm relaxes, the pressure in the thorax (chest area) is pushed up and the air rushes out.

The air breathed in contains oxygen, which passes into the millions of alveoli in the lungs. These hold tiny cells of air which give off the oxygen into the tiny blood vessels called capillaries, which transport it into the bloodstream. At the same time carbon dioxide is extracted from the blood and subsequently expelled through the mouth and nose.

Breath is life, and we owe it to ourselves to breathe more deeply, to give ourselves plenty of fresh air and to protect our lungs from the damage caused by cigarette smoke and chemical pollution. Reflexologists can often tell if a person smokes because the lung reflexes have a granular feel. Many are able to tell if a person smoked even many years before, because the bottom of the lungs still has sensitive reflex points which may identify a dormant residue of tar in the lungs.

Most adults breathe over 13,000 litres of air a day and, although the body can survive for days without water and weeks without food, we would be dead in a few minutes without air. Every minute we breathe in and out about fifteen times.

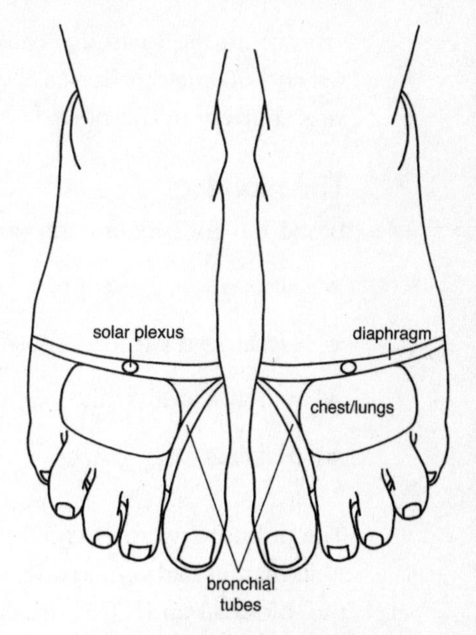

Position of respiratory reflexes on the feet

How reflexology and VRT help

VRT and reflexology can help increase the lung capacity by stimulating the diaphragm to contract and relax fully. Asthma and bronchitis respond well to VRT, as the top of the foot can be worked vigorously to help desensitise or decongest the lungs.

The cardiovascular and circulatory system

The heart

The heart is the central muscle in the cardiovascular and circulatory system and is vital for life. Its role is to pump oxygen and the nutrients required by the body to every cell and tissue. Positioned slightly left of centre in the thoracic cavity, the heart is the size of a small fist and weighs about 255g. In twenty-four hours the heart pumps about 36,000 litres of blood round the body.

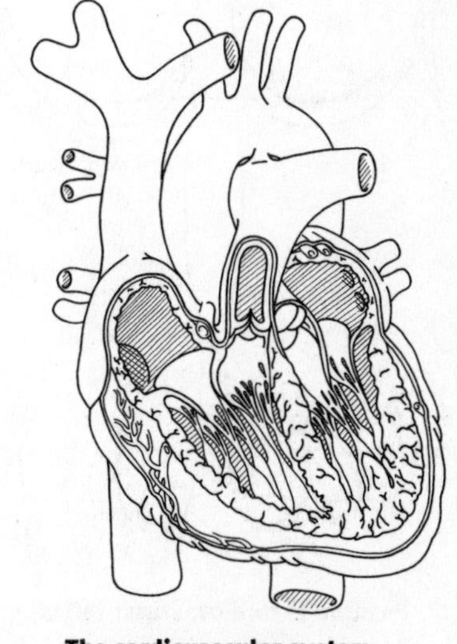

The cardiovascular system

The heart has four chambers: the right and left atria (upper) and the right and left ventricles (lower). Blood vessels that take oxygenated blood away from the heart are called arteries. They are large, elastic tubes which become smaller as they stretch further away. The aorta is the largest artery in the body.

The blood

Blood has four main components:

- plasma
- erythrocytes (red corpuscles)
- lymphocytes (white corpuscles)
- platelets.

The pulmonary artery carries blood from the heart to the lungs, where it discharges carbon dioxide and picks up oxygen to be carried through the bloodstream. This freshly oxygenated blood carries nutrients throughout the body, by means of arteries and capillaries, to the cells. The veins carry carbon dioxide and waste back to the heart and lungs to be discharged.

How reflexology and VRT help

One of the key factors in reflexology is that it improves the circulation, and in doing so increases the vitality of the body. The circulatory system is the front line for maintaining the body's immunity. Since it is fighting potential disease all the time, it is essential that antibodies are directed to vulnerable areas in the body. A sluggish system means that the circulation is below par. With VRT the heart reflexes and the entire dorsal area (the whole body) should be worked thoroughly to stimulate the circulation and increase immunity to disease. New VRT heart reflexes on the ankle help balance the entire cardiovascular system.

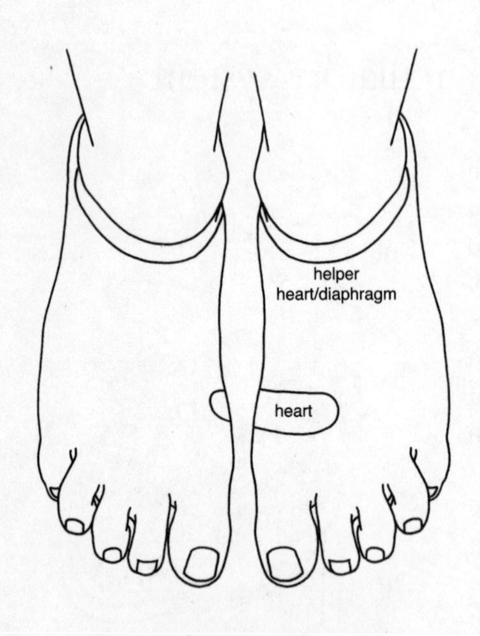

Position of cardiovascular reflexes on the feet

The digestive system

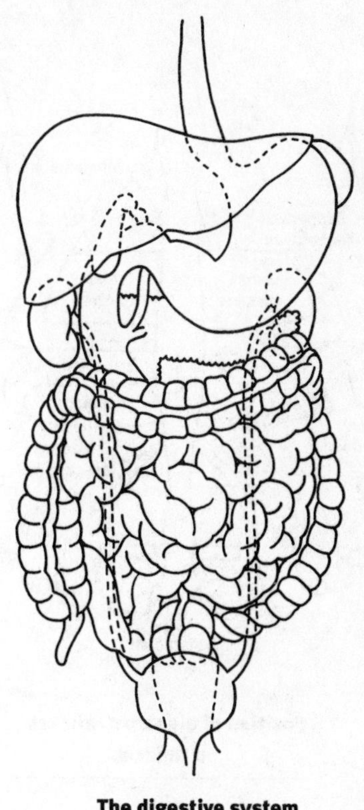

The digestive system

This system converts food into substances that the body is able to absorb and use for energy and heat. It begins at the mouth where the food is chewed (masticated) by thirty-two teeth with the help of saliva and the tongue. The pharynx passes the food to the stomach via the oesophagus and from there it travels to the small intestine, which is made up of the duodenum, jejunum and the ileum where most of the digestive processes take place. The liver, gall bladder and pancreas also aid digestion. The waste matter passes into the large intestine (bowel) via the ileo-caecal valve, which prevents it going backwards, from where it is expelled via the rectum and anus.

The colon is divided into sections as it curves its way round the abdomen: the ascending colon passes up the right side of the abdomen, turns left to become the transverse colon, and then down to become the descending colon. At a sharp bend near the end of the colon it becomes the rectum, which leads to the anus, the point of exit from the body.

How reflexology and VRT help

The body needs optimum nutrition to function properly; if the digestive system is impaired, the rest of the body suffers. Many naturopaths treat the bowel first regardless of the patient's symptoms, because they maintain that the rest of the body cannot recover until the digestion is improved. Some books on the care of the colon describe in vivid detail the inner state of some people's digestive systems, where waste matter festers in unhealthy bowels that are unable to discharge it all. Reflexologists are trained to work carefully over the entire intestinal area, and tender reflexes will often highlight areas in the abdomen where pain or bloating are felt. By working these areas the digestive

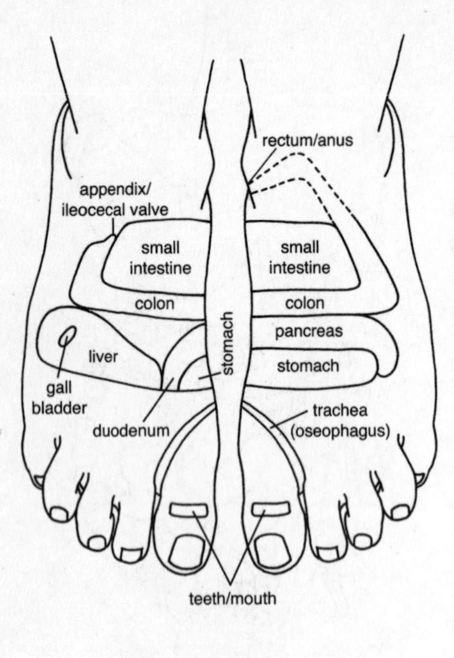

Position of digestive reflexes on the feet

system can be stimulated to work more effectively.

If the person treated is constipated, the reflexes of the bowel can feel harder to a reflexologist and slightly bruised to the client. If diarrhoea is the problem, the reflexes can feel softer to the therapist but prickly to the client as there is often a degree of inflammation in the bowel. VRT and reflexology work towards normalising the body functions, and the same reflexes are worked whether the bowels are too active or not active enough. VRT and Synergistic Reflexology are extremely successful at treating irritable bowel, but lasting success is achieved when dietary habits are addressed at the same time.

The urinary system

This system comprises the two kidneys, the ureters which transport urine to the bladder, and the urethra which in turn passes the urine out of the body.

The kidneys

Kidneys are bean-shaped and measure about 10cm x 5cm x 2.5cm. They are situated at the back of the body in the area of the waistline, and the right kidney is slightly lower than the left. The kidneys are the master chemists of the body: their function is to separate waste products from the blood and to keep it chemically balanced despite the variations in food and liquids consumed. Much of the water, salts, glucose and some urea are returned to the bloodstream, but the waste and excess becomes urine. Up to 180 litres of fluid are processed daily by the kidneys, and 1.5 litres is excreted by the body as urine.

The ureters are thin muscular tubes, up to 30cm long, that carry urine from the kidneys to the bladder, which is a very elastic, muscular sac with a capacity of 600ml or more. When the bladder is full we feel an urge to urinate and the urine is consciously released via the urethra, a narrow muscular tube only 4cm long in a woman and 20cm long in a man.

How reflexology and VRT help

Reflexologists work all the reflexes of the urinary system to help it function efficiently. VRT has proved extremely effective in helping cystitis, bladder infections and pelvic floors weakened by childbirth and resulting in stress incontinence. Several reports have been received of kidney stones being passed naturally after receiving VRT, reflexology or both. The kidney reflexes on the dorsum and the plantar of the feet can often feel tender but can be worked vigorously to stimulate the function of the entire urinary system.

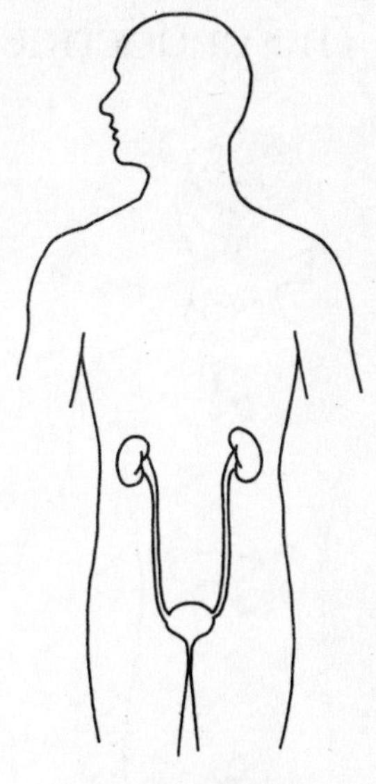

The urinary system

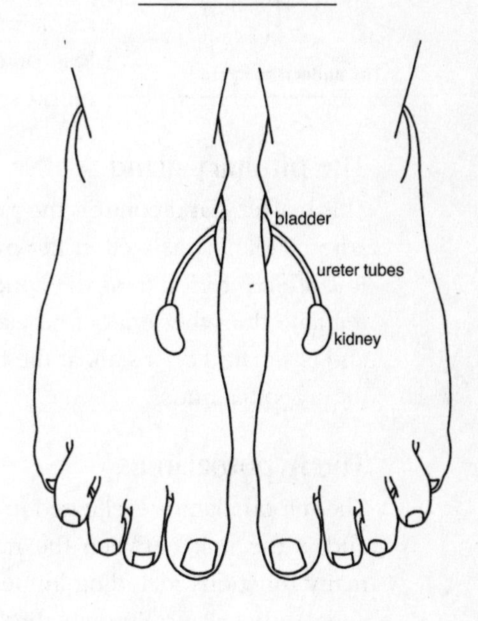

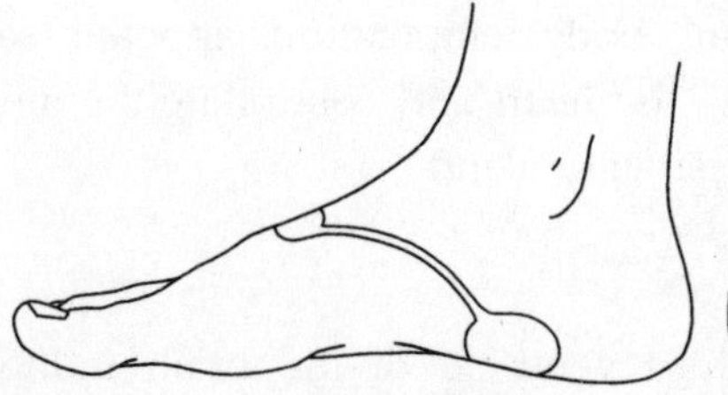

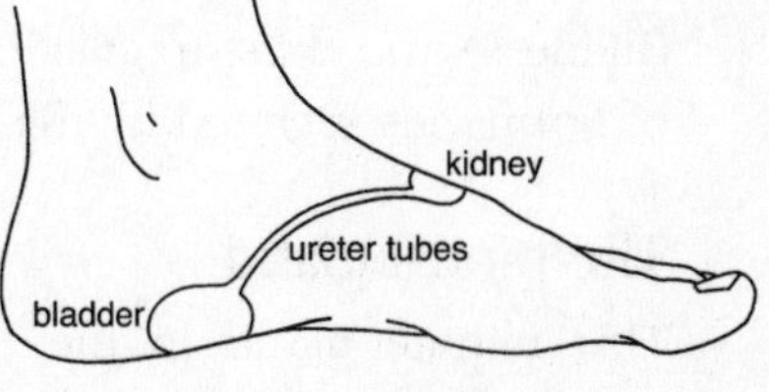

Position of urinary reflexes on the feet

The endocrine system

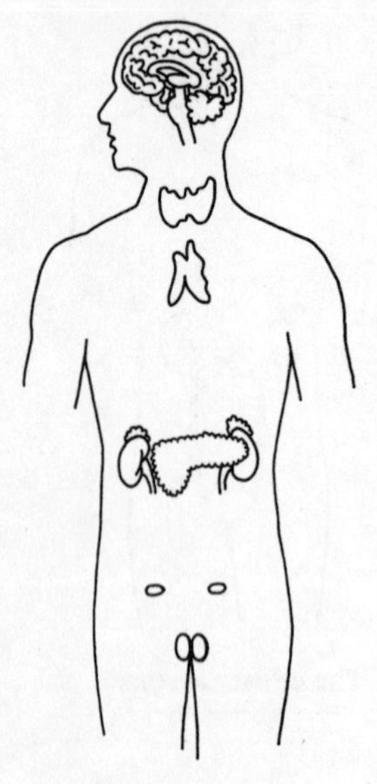

The endocrine system

This, the hormonal system of the body, regulates the many metabolic processes and is essential for regulating the body's chemical functions. The endocrine gland secretions work to control changes in the body, including growth rate and sexual functions. Endocrine glands are ductless glands that secrete hormones into the bloodstream. These are then carried round until they reach the part of the body targeted to respond to a particular hormone. These glands function independently, but require a general hormonal balance in the body in order to function properly. The slightest irregularity in hormonal output can result in major differences ranging from hair loss or excessive growth to lack of libido or mood swings.

The pituitary gland

This master gland controls the pineal, thyroid, thymus, parathyroid and adrenal glands, as well as the ovaries, testes and part of the pancreas. It is often referred to as the conductor of the orchestra, as its role is to regulate the other endocrine glands. The pituitary is the size of a pea and is situated on a stalk at the base of the brain. It works closely with the hypothalamus.

The hypothalamus

The hypothalamus is situated in the third ventricle (cavity) of the brain and is the link between the nervous and endocrine systems. It has many functions including influence on our sexual behaviour, and has centres that determine whether something is painful or pleasant. It is also responsible for controlling body temperature, appetite, satiety (fullness) and thirst, regulating the heart and controlling the amount of hormones secreted by the pituitary gland.

The pineal gland

This minute gland in the third ventricle of the brain influences behaviour and mood swings and secretes melatonin, which is believed to be a light receptor. The correct amount of melatonin is essential for our body-clocks to work properly. Conversely too much of this hormone produces sleep and lethargy. It is now thought that the body cannot always produce enough melatonin to ensure sleep if it has been exposed to too much light. In the USA and certain other countries melatonin is sold in capsule form to promote sleep in cases of insomnia and to regulate the body's sleep patterns when flying and thus to prevent jet-lag.

The thymus gland

Located in the upper chest, is part of the lymphatic system, but is also an endocrine gland which contains T-lymphocytes that help the body defend itself against disease (see p. 41).

The thyroid and parathyroid glands

These glands are in the front and base of the neck. The thyroid is the largest of all the glands and controls growth and metabolism in the body through the secretion of thyroxine. Metabolism refers to the speed at which the body burns food and utilises its cells, and the thyroid stimulates the rate of all body tissues except the brain and lymph tissues. It is also the storage site in the body for the chemical iodine, which is an essential constituent of thyroxine.

Hyperthyroidism

This refers to an overactive thyroid which produces too much hormone. This results in loss of weight, rapid heartbeat, nervousness and anxiety, and in extreme cases to prominent eyes and a swelling in the neck called a goitre.

Hypothyroidism

Hypothyroidism is much more common than hyperthyroidism and refers to an underactive thyroid which results in weight gain, a dry, flaky skin, lack of energy and general sluggishness and lack of concentration. Many women have mild symptoms of hyperthyroidism and yet blood tests show that their hormonal levels are within the normal range. VRT and reflexology can help to stimulate and balance the thyroid gland if it is under- or overproducing.

The parathyroid glands

These consist of between three and ten minute glands embedded in the connective tissue of the thyroid. They secrete a hormone which regulates the calcium levels in the blood and the tissue fluid. Calcium builds and strengthens the bones as well as aiding the nervous system and maintaining the correct pH balance in the blood.

The adrenal or suprarenal glands

These are situated on top of each kidney but have a totally separate function from the kidneys. Each gland has an outer portion called the cortex, which is essential to life as it synthesises over thirty different steroids. Steroid hormones control and balance various chemicals in the body, convert carbohydrates to glucogen in the liver and influence sexual development and behaviour. The cortex releases sex hormones into the body as well as a substance called aldosterone, which regulates much of the mineral and water content of the body by stimulating the kidneys. The medulla plays an important role in stimulating the sympathetic nervous system as it releases adrenalin and noradrenalin into the body to help the body respond to threatening situations. These hormones increase the metabolic rate and make the person more alert so that they can deal with a 'fight or flight' situation. Overwork or stress can trigger the body to keep producing too much adrenalin, leading to adrenal exhaustion.

The pancreas

The pancreas contains the islets of Langerhans, which secrete insulin to regulate the level of blood sugar and convert its heat into energy. Insulin converts glucose to glycogen and aids the synthesis of DNA and RNA. Glucose is the main source of energy for all our body cells and glycogen helps stimulate the liver to raise the glucose levels in the blood. DNA is the hereditary gene material in each cell and specifies every aspect of a person's genetic coding. RNA acts as its manager – between them they provide the coding instructions for protein synthesis. The pancreas is also part of the digestive system (see p. 45) as it produces digestive enzymes.

The ovaries and testes

These are also part of the reproductive system, described on p. 56. The ovaries produce oestrogen and progesterone while the testes

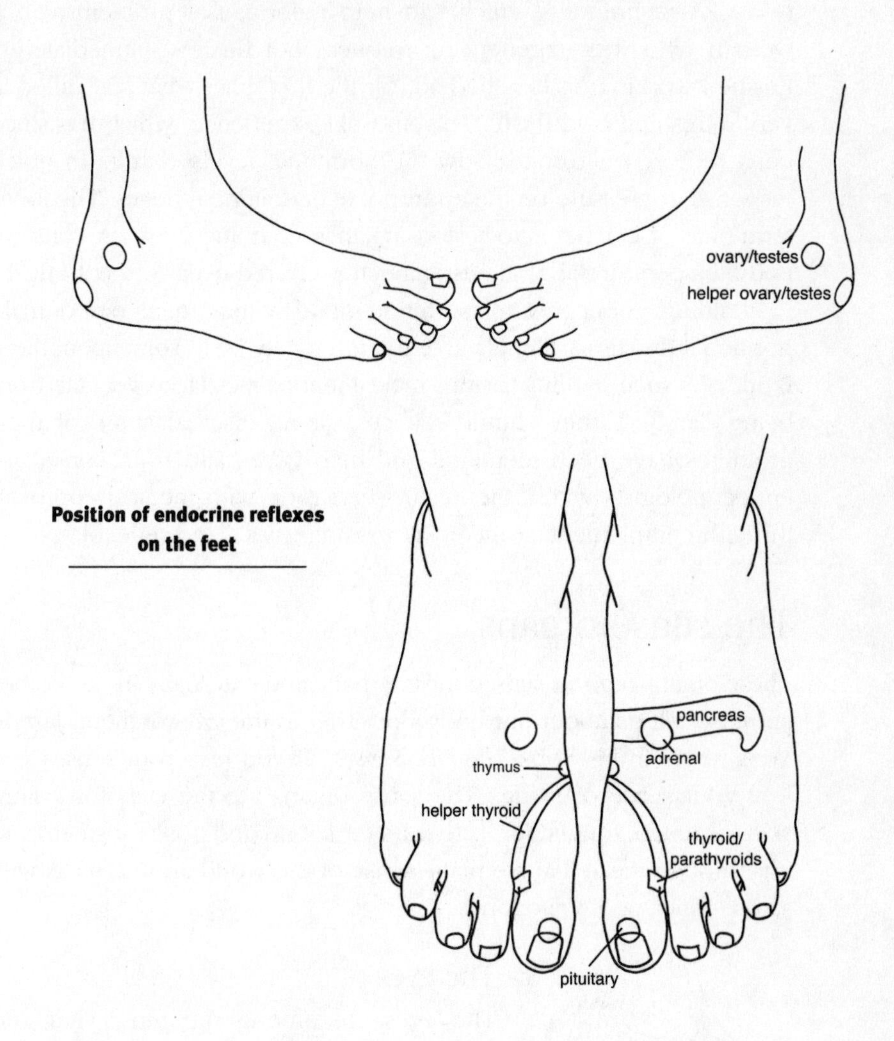

Position of endocrine reflexes on the feet

manufacture sperm and contain cells that manufacture testosterone, the hormone that produces male characteristics.

How reflexology and VRT help

VRT, and reflexology in general, balance the body by triggering the organs and glands to work to their optimum ability. The hormonal system therefore responds extremely well to gentle pressure on the reflexes; the new VRT helper ovary point on the base of the heel and the 'pituitary pinch' appear to accelerate the body's response to normalise the secretion of hormones. At a seminar I demonstrated these two VRT techniques, which can help menopausal problems, on a woman who was experiencing frequent hot flushes. Immediately I finished working on her she had, for the first time, what she called 'a very refreshing cold flush'. This unusual experience, which has since been repeated, illustrates how the hormonal levels change in quick response to pressure on the appropriate endocrine reflexes. The long-term aim, of course, is to restore balance or homeostasis. A constant body temperature at all times is much preferred even to a cold flush!

Balding, going grey and suffering mood swings are all part of male hormonal functions. Unpalatable though it may be to some men, there is indeed such a thing as the male menopause! However, far from being daunted, they should rejoice – it means that some of their problems have been identified and help is at hand from consultant endocrinologists within the health service or, with medical approval, through complementary medicine including VRT and reflexology.

The sense organs

These organs register sensations internally and externally in our bodies and also tell us about our body's position in the environment. Jan de Vries writes in his book *The Five Senses*, 'If you lose your senses you lose your sense of living.' The sense organs are the eyes for vision, skin for touch, tongue for taste, ears for sound and nose for smell, and it is through these that we make sense of the world around us as well as our inner bodily workings.

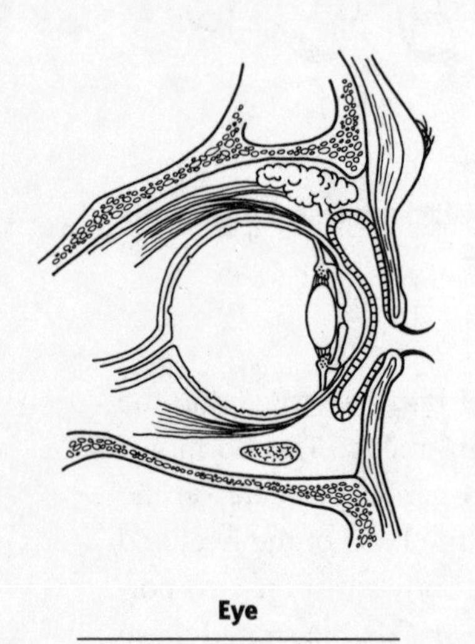

Eye

The eyes

The eyes are among the most vital and complex organs of the body. They are protected by bone and fatty tissue in the orbital cavity of the skull, and the optic nerve supplies information to and from the brain. They rotate on three axes, vertical, horizontal and oblique, and depend on the circulation of blood, lymph and nerve messages just like any other organ. The eyes which, despite their complexity, move with the use of only six muscles, have three layers of tissue:

- the tough outside layer is the sclera and cornea, which bends the light rays
- the middle vascular layer includes the iris, which regulates the amount of light that enters
- the inner layer is the retina, upon which the lens adjusts the focus. The retina can be easily damaged and even become detached.

For lubrication and cleansing purposes the eyes are continually bathed with fluid from the tear ducts.

The skin

Skin has two layers, the dermis and the epidermis, and it is this material that covers and protects the body.

The dermis is the unseen fatty lower part of the skin and is very tough, being composed of collagen and elastic fibres. All the lymph and blood vessels, hair roots, follicles and glands are contained in the dermis. The nerve endings send messages back to the spinal cord and on to the brain. If we touch a hot pan the nerves send a message to our brain to remove the hand before we are consciously aware of having done so.

We perspire through our skin, and the sweat glands are situated in the dermis along with the nerve endings that give us the vital information about touch and temperature. These glands are found throughout our body but are concentrated in the feet, groin and armpit. The use of antiperspirants actually restricts the body in carrying out its vital task of cleansing and cooling the entire system; it is also advisable to avoid deodorants that contain aluminium, which is toxic.

The epidermis is the top layer of skin, the part that comes into contact with the outside world. It forms a protective layer over the nerve endings and sebaceous glands and keeps water and foreign bodies out, unless it is injured or perforated in some way. Hairs and perspiration pass through the epidermis from the dermis. The epidermis is a barometer of our general health and reflects what is going on internally. A poor digestion will result in a pallid skin and possibly spots and blemishes. Ageing is inevitable, but drinking plenty of pure water and eating the right kinds of food can help preserve the epidermis and slow down the thinning of the skin and loss of elasticity.

The tongue

The tongue helps us to taste, swallow and speak. It is a voluntary muscle covered in papillae which contain nine thousand taste buds, situated mainly at the back of the tongue. These taste buds recognise four basic tastes – salty, bitter, sweet and sour – and the tongue's role when we are eating or drinking is to relay the chemical content of the substance to the brain through nerve impulses. To gather all the information that the body requires for safe consumption of food, it works closely in conjunction with the eyes and the nose.

The tongue is also essential to speech. Anyone who has had a mild anaesthetic injection from a dentist will realise how difficult it is to speak when the tongue is partially paralysed!

The ears

These are a complex three-part mechanism in the head that not only provides the means to hear but also gives balance to the entire body.

The external ear – the visible part attached to the side of the head – is called the auricle. Its function is to collect sound waves and conduct them to the external auditory canal, which also contains the glands that secrete wax to lubricate the ear mechanism.

The middle ear is also known as the tympanic cavity or eardrum, and it is here that the sound is amplified. The sound waves hit the

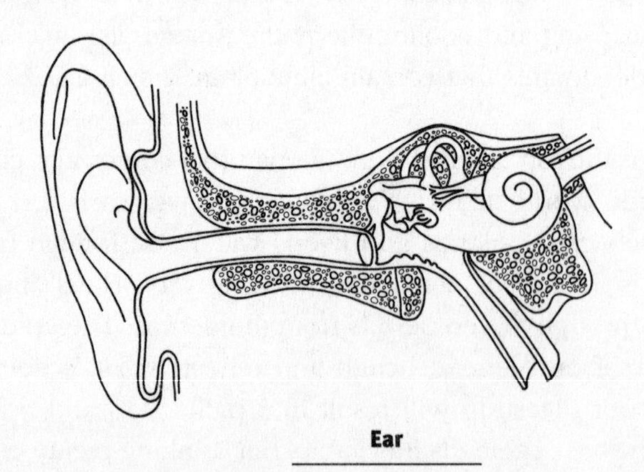

Ear

eardrum, and the bones in the middle ear, known as the anvil, hammer and stirrup, magnify the vibration. The Eustachian (auditory) tube is a narrow tube that connects the middle ear with the nasopharynx to ensure that the air pressure in the middle ear is the same as the atmospheric pressure. The middle ear is often prone to infection in children, and it is this part of the ear that *pops* when the air pressure changes in an aeroplane, for example.

The inner ear or labyrinth is concerned with the equilibrium or balance of the body, and transmits vibrations to the cochlea which is the essential organ of hearing. It is the channel that transmits information to the brain via the eighth cranial nerve.

'My children have ear problems including frequent infections, glue ear and a perforated eardrum. Is there a general, easy VRT treatment I could learn to help them?'

The ear reflexes can feel quite tender and, although no child welcomes real pain, if they are already suffering they may be agreeably surprised when their earache subsides fast after VRT. It is advisable to take children to a professional reflexologist, who can show you the key reflexes to work between treatments. Train your children to locate a particularly tender spot on the ear reflexes at the base of the fingers, and to rub it firmly when the hand is palm down, and weight-bearing, on a table.

The nose

The nose is the organ that controls the sense of smell, also referred to as the olfactory sense. The nose is able to recognise thousands of different smells and relay the information to the brain via special sensory receptors in the nasal cavity. It is also part of the respiratory system (see p. 42). Air inhaled through the nose is filtered and warmed before it reaches the lungs.

The nose is at the front line for removing toxins before they penetrate the body. It is lined with a hairy mucous membrane containing blood vessels that are close to the surface. The three pairs of sinuses branch out from the nasal passages and go into the skull. Nasal

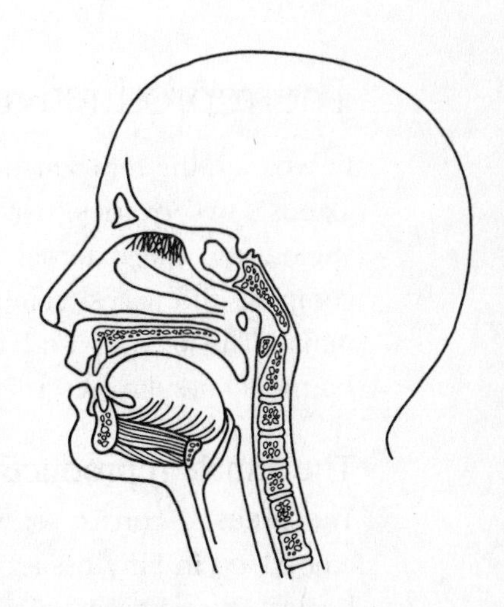

Nasal passages and mouth

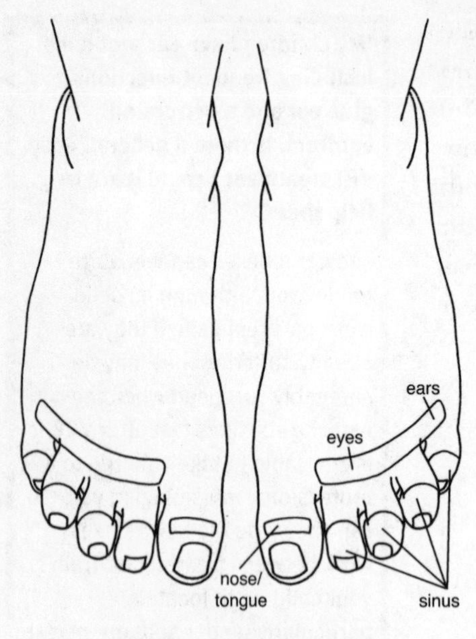

Position of sensory reflexes on the feet

infections can sometimes spread into the sinuses and even into the entire respiratory system.

How reflexology and VRT can help

Both techniques are extremely effective at pinpointing and treating the sense organs. The eyes, ears, nose and tongue reflexes can all be found on the fingers and thumbs as well as on the toes. On the hands they are easy to access for self-help techniques, and the reflexes will often feel extremely sore if the person has a sinus problem or toothache. There are minute reflexes round the big toe and thumb that relate to the nose and mouth and respond especially well to the firm pressure of VRT on a standing foot.

The skin can sometimes become a little blemished when you begin a series of reflexology treatments. The body will be stimulated to throw off toxins, and one of the main vehicles of elimination is the skin.

The reproductive system

In women, the reproductive system consists of the breasts (mammary glands), two ovaries, two fallopian tubes, the uterus, the cervix, the vagina and the external genitalia. In men the reproductive organs comprise the testes, seminal vesicles, *vas deferens*, prostate and the penis. The ovaries and testes also form part of the endocrine or hormonal system (see p. 48).

The female reproductive system

The breasts consist of fifteen to twenty milk-producing glands embedded in fatty tissue. Their function is to supply milk to nourish babies. During pregnancy hormonal changes take place in the breasts: prolactin and oxytocin are secreted, which results in breast milk being produced and released within hours of a mother giving birth. Men have breasts too, but they are undeveloped.

The ovaries also form part of the endocrine system (see p. 48) and are the female reproductive glands. A baby girl is born with about forty thousand eggs in her ovaries and from puberty, when she begins menstruating, to the menopause at about the age of fifty she will release one egg or ovum a month. Occasionally more than one egg is produced and, if fertilised, can produce multiple births. At the middle of the monthly cycle the egg travels down the fallopian tube (or uterine tube). If that egg is not fertilised in this tube by a sperm, the lining of the uterus will be shed two weeks later, as the monthly period, because it is not needed to nourish a growing embryo. The pituitary gland controls the function of the ovaries, and the hypothalamus also plays a role in stimulating the secretion of hormones that play vital roles in the monthly cycle.

The uterus is the muscular organ in which a baby develops, and is situated in the middle of the pelvis with the bladder in front and the rectum behind. The top of the uterus is called the fundus, the middle the body and the lowest part the cervix. The cervix leads into the vagina, a hollow muscular organ that connects the uterus to the external genitalia which include the vulva and clitoris. The extremely elastic vagina is capable of expanding to receive the penis during intercourse and to let a baby pass through at birth.

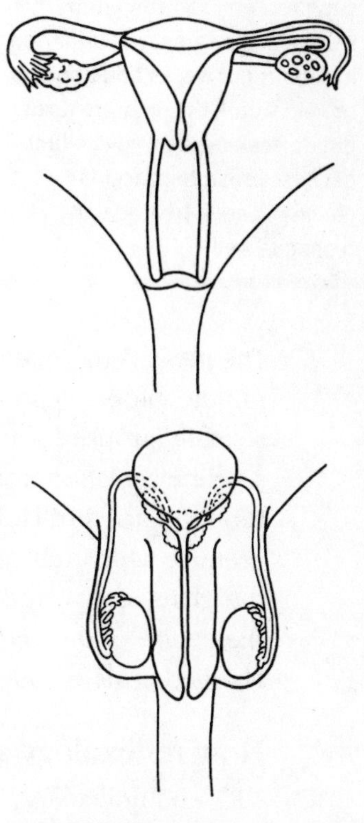

The male (above) and female (top) reproductive systems

The male reproductive system

The testes are two sex glands that descend from the abdominal cavity while a boy baby is still in the womb, and by the eighth month have reached the external pouch of skin called the scrotum. The testicles produce the hormone testosterone and sperm, which mature for three weeks in the epididymis, a coiled tube lying round the testes. Each sex gland is attached to the body by a single cord called the *vas deferens* (sperm duct), which contains a number of nerves and blood vessels. The sperm then travels to the seminal vesicles, which produce seminal fluid. When a man has an orgasm his sperm passes into the urethra and is ejaculated with the seminal fluid. The bladder and testicles share the same exit, the 20cm urethra which runs the length of the penis. A muscular action prevents urine and seminal fluids being passed at the same time.

'I am fifty-seven and have an enlarged prostate gland which causes me to urinate frequently, especially at night. Can VRT help?'

It is extremely effective, particularly in conjunction with specially formulated nutritional supplements. VRT can often reduce the frequency of urination in a matter of weeks and appears to help shrink the prostate itself, but do seek medical advice first because prostate cancer is common and, if treated early, responds well.

The prostate gland is a cluster of small glands which surround the urethra at the point where it joins the bladder. There is some debate about the actual function of the prostate: it is suggested that it provides additional secretions into the seminal fluid to help the active movement of the sperm. Many men's prostate glands begin to enlarge and stiffen after the age of forty-five, and in later life this can put pressure on the urethra that it surrounds. The first sign of prostate trouble is a weakened flow of urine with an urgent need to pass water at night even though both flow and contents are low.

The penis is the male sex organ and consists of spongy tissue full of minute blood vessels which become engorged when the man is sexually aroused, causing it to become erect and increase in size. A single ejaculation contains millions of sperm, only one of which is required to fertilise the woman's egg. The penis surrounds the urethra, which transports the semen and urine. The tip of the penis, the glans, is covered by a loose hood of skin called the foreskin. In the centre of the glans is a slit from which urine and semen are discharged. This is called the external urethral orifice.

How reflexology and VRT can help

VRT and reflexology have a very positive role to play in supporting a healthy reproductive system. The endocrine system can be worked to help regulate the production of particular hormones. There are reflexes

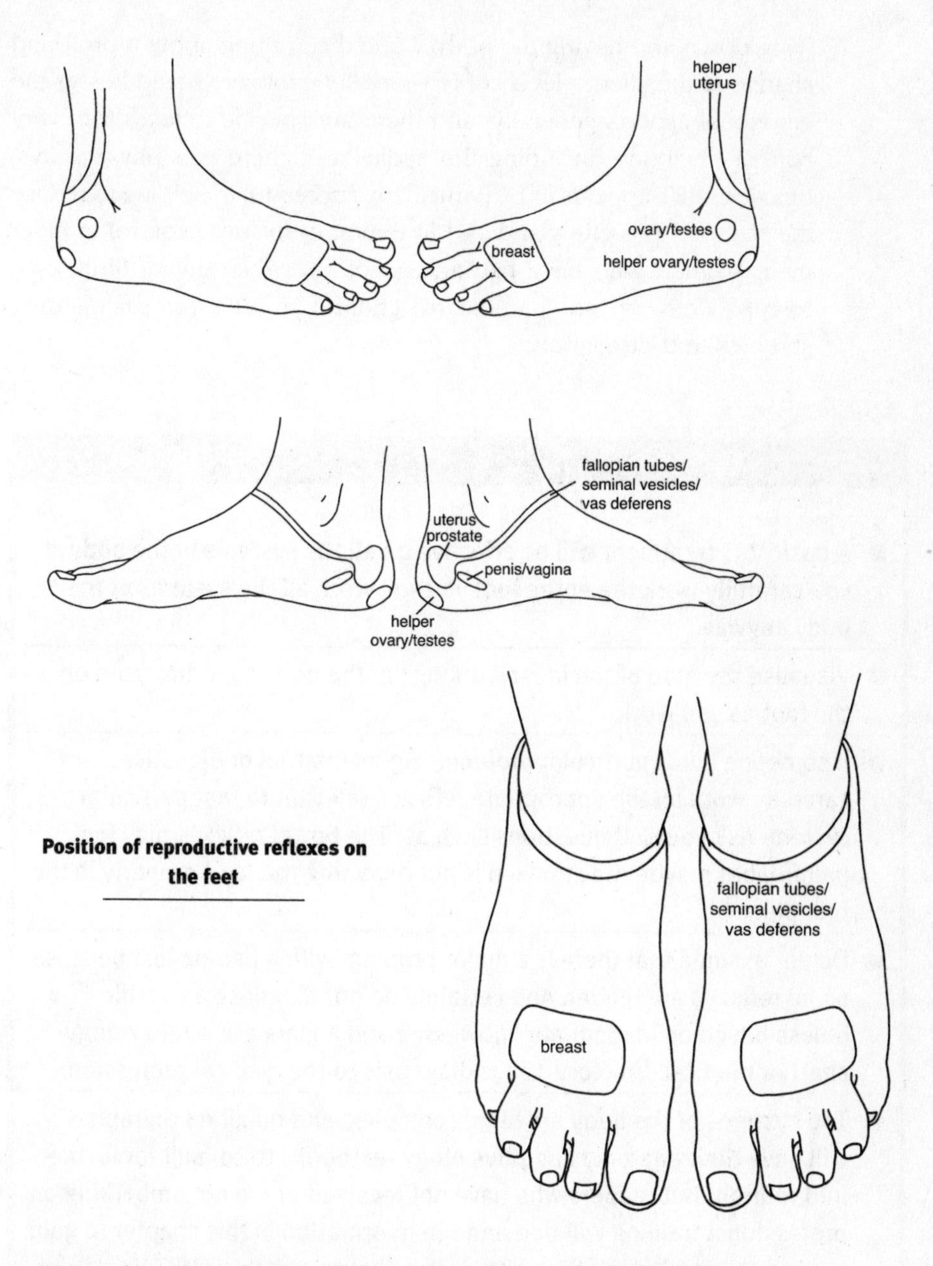

Position of reproductive reflexes on the feet

connected with every part of the reproductive system, and reflexology has a major role to play in regulating a woman's menstrual cycle as well as helping to improve prostate problems in men and sexual difficulties in both sexes. Reflexology is a gentle, relaxing therapy, and often clients will confide that they are too wound up, too tired or just too plain disinterested to have sex with their partner. The time spent lying down and having the body worked can bring about a profound change in the client's levels of tension. Reflexology also addresses the emotional aspects generally, and there are specific reflexes for every part of the body, including the genitalia, if there is a physical dysfunction. VRT appears to be particularly successful in helping to reduce the size of a prostate gland and in toning up bladder control in older men. Women who have had an episiotomy when giving birth, or a forceps delivery, are particularly grateful to VRT for easing their soreness and discomfort.

Key points to remember

- A basic VRT treatment will be effective on all the systems of the body. If you carefully work the entire foot you will work all the systems of the body anyway.
- Visualise the map of the inner workings of the body superimposed on the foot as you work.
- If someone has a particular problem, e.g. menstrual or digestive, carefully work all the appropriate reflexes relevant to that particular system. Ask yourself questions such as: The bowel reflexes may feel painful, but maybe the stomach is not digesting the food properly in the first place?
- Do not assume that there is a major problem with a person just because some reflexes are tender. And certainly do not diagnose a specific illness based on inadequate knowledge and a glance at a reflexology chart or medical directory. Leave diagnosis to the medical profession.
- The systems of the body are highly complex, and qualified therapists will have their anatomy and physiology textbooks to consult for further information. But readers who have not received or are not embarking on professional training will find enough information in this chapter to gain a working knowledge of the body when they give a Basic VRT treatment.

Who can be treated, and how

The three VRT treatment options

VRT WORKS EXTREMELY WELL ON ITS OWN AS A BRIEF FOUR- OR FIVE-MINUTE treatment, but ideally it should be incorporated into the start and finish of a conventional session. This way it consolidates and enhances the standard treatment given to a person who is lying or sitting down. The versatility of VRT and its powerful techniques also allows the therapist a third option: a comprehensive but shortened reflexology treatment that takes about twenty minutes called Complete VRT. Here the reflexes on the sole of the feet are quickly worked for about ten minutes, with a few minutes of VRT, including some specialised techniques, before and afterwards. This arrangement does not give the person so long to relax, but can be as effective as a full treatment. One of the more amusing aspects of teaching VRT is the gasps of surprise from people who find they can relax and even feel comfortable while their feet are worked as they stand!

Conventional reflexology always starts with a series of relaxation techniques to loosen the feet and generally allow the person being treated to unwind. The gentle massaging and pressure on the feet stimulates the reflexes generally, so that they are ready to respond when the reflexologist begins to work the specific pressure reflexes. With VRT this may at first appear to be incompatible, as the client has to lie down before the feet can be worked. But it is important to learn and apply the relaxation techniques because they can loosen up the feet before you begin to work them in the standing position.

The three treatment options all achieve excellent results, so you can be flexible in your approach depending on the time available and the needs of a particular person. However, it is not realistic for professional therapists to offer *very* short individual treatments, although many reflexologists are often asked how much they would charge for one after a national newspaper wrote about VRT as 'Three-minute Magic'! The shortest viable treatment in a clinic or private practice would be about twenty minutes.

- Excellent results can be obtained by treating clients once or twice per week with these new techniques, and I generally combine VRT with three-quarters of an hour of conventional reflexology.
- Larger groups of people can be treated with a twenty- or thirty-minute session each using the shortened Complete VRT. This method opens up enormous possibilities for treating in a short space of time groups of people such as office workers, hospice patients and sports teams.
- A group booking of, say, a sports team, musicians or dancers could be made on a weekly basis and a reflexologist would give them all a five-minute Basic VRT treatment.

Reflexologists have a great advantage over many complementary therapists because the feet and hands are very accessible parts of the body. No implements, needles or even a therapy couch need be used, and only the footwear is removed. In the case of Vertical Reflex Therapy, it takes only a few minutes while the person is standing and can be performed anywhere! Reports have come to me of VRT being administered in many unusual places such as parties, in the office, on a cricket pitch, at a PTA meeting, a classical concert, on the beach, a cycle track and even on an aeroplane.

'How many VRT treatments do you need before you see results?'

Everyone is different in their response. VRT, however, often works very quickly – you may see results straight after your first five-minute treatment. Equally, do not give up if, after regular weekly or twice-weekly treatments, you experience no improvement for three or four weeks. If there is still no effect, you may need a different therapy altogether. It has usually taken some time for the body to become ill, so it will often take a while for that person to recover.

The five-minute Basic VRT treatment

Some of the most impressive VRT successes have been achieved after only a few minutes' work; all the important reflexes of the body, and subsequent fine-tuning techniques, can be included even in this brief session. Don't look on five-minute

Case study

A few years ago three reflexologists were returning from a conference in Finland where they had heard me present a paper on VRT. Their plane was delayed by several hours and when they finally took off all the passengers were decidedly tired and rather fractious and one of the reflexologists complained that her back was aching. The other two decided to put the new VRT techniques they had learnt into practice and worked on her standing feet as she stood in the aisle of the plane. Soon a crowd of young men from another conference were queuing up and received VRT on their feet. The stewards and hostesses were intrigued but did not feel that company policy would allow them to take their shoes off, so they stood while their hands were worked! They then felt so relaxed that they lay back in the seats, while the young men, suitably revitalised, served the free compensatory drinks to the other passengers!

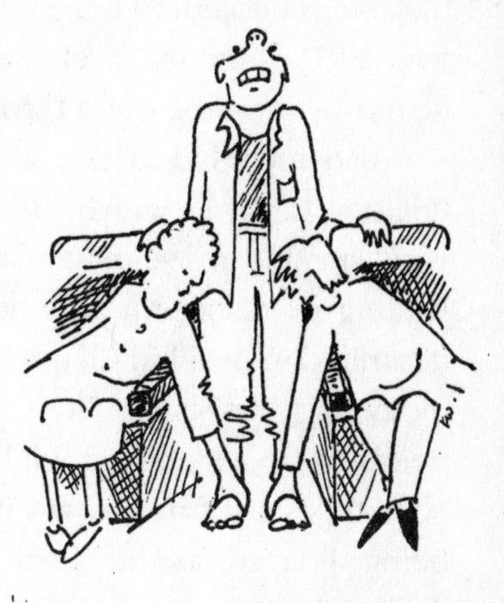

Courtesy Kristine Walker

Basic VRT as just first aid – it has a major role to play in helping family and friends to get well and stay well, and is a valuable method of self-help reflexology. It is also used by other therapists such as osteopaths, aromatherapists and masseurs to consolidate their own type of treatment. Although reflexologists are more likely to offer the shortened twenty-minute Complete VRT described below, they might offer blocks of five-minute Basic VRT treatments to groups of people in sports teams, schools and physiotherapy units. One practitioner I taught normally went to the football club changing rooms to give post-match reflexology to the team. After training in VRT she is now able to give the players a short VRT booster on the touchline at matches as well.

The twenty-minute comprehensive Complete VRT treatment

A VRT student once stopped me at a conference and told me how helpful my reflexology sandwich had been to her practice. I was puzzled until she explained that she used 'a thin slice of VRT either side of bigger chunk of reflexology'! This treatment incorporates all the VRT techniques, but the person being treated can also benefit from some relaxation movements and ten minutes of reflexology on the sole of the foot. This shortened treatment is a major breakthrough. Many therapists just do not believe they can treat the soles of the feet in only ten minutes, but it is pertinent to remember that the rest of the foot has already been worked. This is because the brief working of the sole is enough to trigger a powerful reflex response when coupled with VRT, as the main reflexes on the plantar have already been stimulated by working them through the top of the feet.

Also included is the soothing technique known as Diaphragm Rocking (DR), in which the feet are gently rocked in a relaxing but very specific movement which allows the body to pump energy, healing or relaxation to where it is most needed. The technique is described in detail in Chapter 7. It forms a profound addition to reflexology as it assists the body in prioritising where the healing energy needs to be channelled while the person is in the reclining position. Sometimes DR can give an indication of exactly where the energy is being directed, as the client will feel a rush of warmth or tingling in the weakest part of their body.

This shortened treatment gives all the healing benefits of a full session because it is so powerful, but the client does miss out on the longer period of peace and relaxation that he or she would

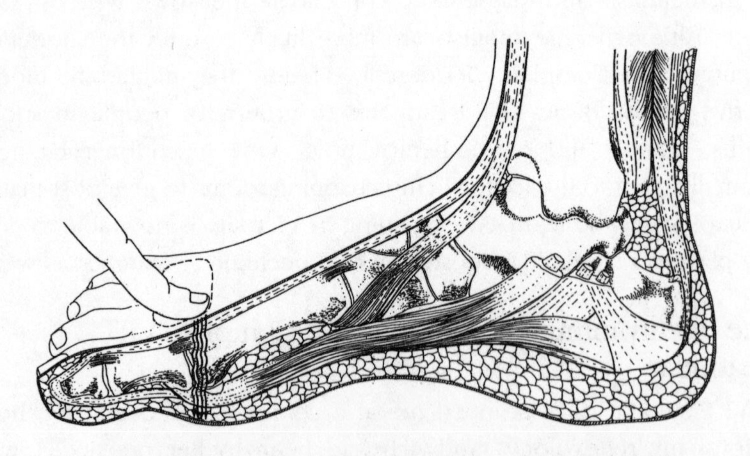

Cross-section of foot showing penetration of reflex layers

Case study

Agile, fifteen-year-old Nicky is an excellent gymnast who had landed awkwardly after sliding down a rope. Her lower lumbar area was extremely tender, with sharp pain whenever she leaned backwards. I briefly worked her feet with five-minute Basic VRT and found the spinal reflexes very tender on both feet. Then I worked synergistically on her hands and feet hip reflexes before finding the Zonal Trigger for the lumbar area. I asked her to sit on a chair and place both feet on my lap while I gave her a couple of minutes of gentle Diaphragm Rocking on each foot. Halfway through the second foot she experienced a sharp click between her shoulder blades. When she stood up a minute later her back felt free and she could bend painlessly in all directions. It was the Diaphragm Rocking that made the difference here. It allowed the body to select exactly which part of the spine needed realigning, which turned out to be the upper thoracic because it was trying to compensate for the lower back problem.

conventionally receive. Complete VRT has an important role to play when treating sports teams, children, elderly and terminally ill people, as many more clients can be treated in a shorter time. Young children, ME patients and some invalids, for example, cannot cope with more than about a twenty-minute session; Complete VRT enables you to give them a totally effective treatment without tiring or overtreating them.

VRT and conventional reflexology

VRT is now considered by many reflexologists to be an essential additional skill and I would encourage every therapist to incorporate it into their general treatments. Some students who enquire about courses are concerned that they will have to lengthen their normal treatments to include VRT. But this is not so – there is plenty of time in a thirty- to sixty-minute treatment to treat the entire foot and still leave room for a few minutes of essential VRT. If it were not for the wonderful benefits of deep relaxation I would encourage everyone to shorten their combined VRT and conventional treatments to about half an hour, as positive results can be achieved in anything from three to thirty minutes. My own clients still receive, on average, a fifty-minute treatment in which they are given a few minutes of VRT at the beginning and end of their session. Most of my treatments have not shortened because I realise the enormous value in making extra time for ourselves to regain an inner stillness and a deep sense of relaxation. So the golden rule with VRT is to use it at the beginning and/or end of each session, whatever its length, and to cut down the conventional reflexology by five minutes or so to allow time for VRT.

VRT for chronic and acute problems

Chronic illnesses

The word 'chronic' can describe an illness that is possibly fatal, but can also be applied to long-term degenerative illnesses such as arthritis. Asthma sufferers have a chronic illness even if they manage it well with medication, breathing exercises or nutrition. So 'chronic' can refer to a spectrum of complaints from cancer to ongoing catarrh or sinusitis – in fact, to any illness that does not go away.

If someone has had a health problem for a long time it will not usually respond immediately to medication or complementary therapies. This book, and others on reflexology, describes many cases that have defied the doctors' prognosis; they talk of people with stiff limbs who have had them freed in a matter of minutes, or noses that have unblocked in a day after years of congestion. Never limit the scope of VRT, but it is sensible to expect to wait a while as the body heals itself and adjusts at a cellular level, although reflexology can accelerate these processes. It is not realistic for practical or financial reasons to expect a client to attend more than twice a week for treatment. However, many reflexologists will offer two half-hour appointments a week for the first few weeks as the body responds well to the 'little and often' approach. In the case of family and friends, a person with chronic problems could be treated for a few minutes a day, up to a maximum of three times a week.

An important point to remember

Nearly all the new VRT techniques and new reflexes can be used freely on the feet during a conventional treatment. This is because these powerful new skills are effective, but far less intense, when the person is lying down, as the feet are not weight-bearing.

Case study

A reflexologist returned home from a VRT seminar and was eager to put her new-found skills into practice. Her mother-in-law of ninety-two was staying and agreed to have her feet worked for a maximum of two minutes while standing. Very limited in her movements and virtually confined to the house, she had always refused in the past to lie down and have a reflexology treatment, but felt she could just about cope with VRT for a couple of minutes. She commented that the reflexes were quite painful, but slept exceptionally well. When she awoke the next morning she declared that she wanted to go shopping. That afternoon she enjoyed some fruit-picking despite her family's concern that she was overdoing it. She slept well again and continued to enjoy life due to her renewed mobility.

Acute problems

The term 'acute' can refer to the common cold, a twisted ankle or an upset stomach due to overindulgence – in fact any complaint that comes on suddenly and is not expected to last any length of time. Meningitis can be fatal and is also an acute illness, because it comes on so suddenly. Acute cases in hospital are those which have, for example, been rushed in as an emergency with appendicitis, a heart attack or a burst ulcer.

In acute cases, such as a cold or even after childbirth (which, of course, is a condition rather than an illness), it is very effective to give VRT twice a day to stimulate the immune system to help heal and balance the body. If you are treating yourself with self-help techniques, they can be used four or five times a day for a minute or two with great success. But it is not advisable to use VRT too frequently on others, as the body needs time to adjust.

Who can be safely treated with reflexology and VRT?

Most people from tiny babies to octogenarians can benefit from reflexology, as it is a gentle and non-invasive therapy that aims to balance the body naturally. The International Institute of Reflexology founded by Eunice Ingham suggests that no one need be excluded, whereas some schools of reflexology give students a long list of contra-indications. The professional opinions and decisions of individual bodies should be respected, and I would advise reflexologists to follow their own training and only treat conditions with which they feel comfortable. I have treated and helped pregnant women, people with cancer, epileptics, post- and pre-operative patients and clients suffering from infections with a high temperature such as flu. Yet some reflexologists are taught that all these conditions must be avoided.

'Do people ever get negative results after VRT treatment?'

Very rarely, and none in my own experience. VRT may just not have been the right therapy for such people (for instance, the elderly lady who decided not to continue with the Complete VRT trial I conducted in 1997: see p. 187). Of course, what people feel are negative results may be side-effects or a healing crisis (see p. 93) as the body discharges toxins and makes adjustments. If they persevere, they may well see the wished-for improvement.

At one conference I talked to two reflexologists, from a very conservative school, who were concerned about many of the conditions that the other practitioners were happily treating. These two were not even allowed to treat a woman if she was menstruating! As the discussion continued one rather exasperated delegate asked them, 'Who, then, *can* you actually treat?' The answer was, 'Mostly well people,' which caused many a wry smile!

There are many cautions in some textbooks about not treating pregnant women for fear of causing a miscarriage. A famous reflexologist has said on many occasions that, if reflexology has the power to terminate pregnancies, we could all become the most highly paid abortionists in the world! Many women in the first two months of pregnancy do not even know they are pregnant, and gain great benefit from reflexology with no ill-effects.

Far from causing damage, the stimulation of the immune and lymph systems will help detoxify the body whether the client is suffering from cancer at one extreme or sinusitis at the other. It will not spread infection – it will fight it. However, if you are not a qualified reflexologist the conditions listed below are best avoided because professional training is required to treat them properly. Reflexologists support the body in specific ways by working helper areas and by gently treating sensitive reflexes such as the uterus in pregnancy.

Cautions for non-professionals

- Deep vein thrombosis – to be avoided except by professional therapists.
- Varicose veins – treat the person, but do not work directly on the veins. Work the hands if the feet are covered in veins.
- Epilepsy – some professional reflexologists achieve good results with epileptic conditions, but do not try unless you are fully qualified.
- Pregnancy – you can work the feet very gently, but avoid the reproductive reflexes in the first four months. If you are new to reflexology, avoid treating pregnant women altogether during this early period.
- Heart problems – work the feet very gently and brush over the heart reflex so it is touched but not worked. The new helper heart/diaphragm reflexes on the band of the ankle will enable the heart to be helped indirectly but effectively.

Key points to remember

- **Study the contra-indications on pages 68–9 but be willing to give holistic treatments to most ages and conditions.**
- **VRT often produces results after one treatment, but be realistic and only expect to see benefits after several treatments.**
- **Always try and combine VRT with a conventional reflexology session whenever possible.**
- **Qualified reflexologists can now offer effective shorter treatments to sports teams, offices, hospitals, the elderly etc.**
- **Do not be tempted to overwork chronic conditions with VRT. Twice weekly sessions are sufficient.**
- **Acute cases can be treated twice daily with VRT.**
- **Self-help VRT can be administered several times daily.**
- **Every condition can benefit from VRT and reflexology.**

Basic reflexology techniques and charts

IF YOU ARE NEW TO REFLEXOLOGY, THIS CHAPTER WILL GIVE YOU ALL THE guidelines you need for giving a treatment. This chapter will teach you the standard reflexology finger, thumb and relaxation techniques. It also offers you the option of working with your knuckles and a tiny amount of foot cream if you wish. Once you are familiar with these and the general routines described for treating the feet, you can move on to practising Basic VRT in Chapter 5.

Qualified reflexologists will already have the skills required for Vertical Reflex Therapy, but may be interested in developing the use of knuckles and cream if it is unfamiliar to them.

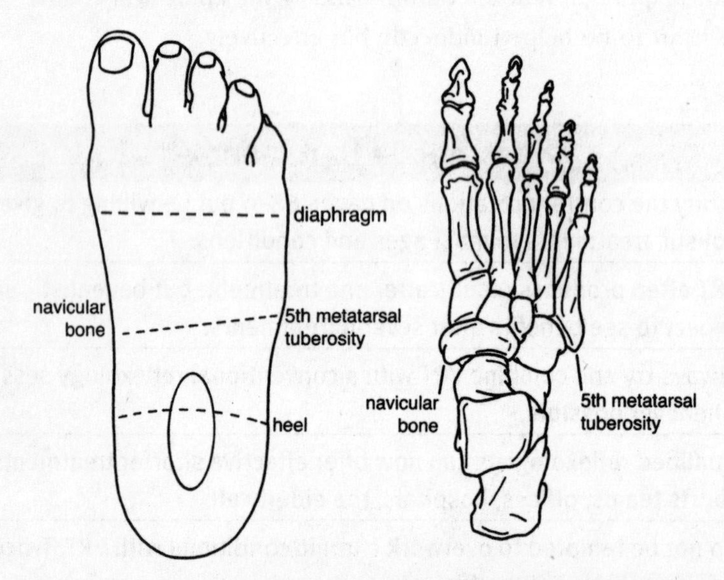

Position of diaphragm/waistline and pelvic girdle on foot

I follow Anthony Porter (ART) and place the waistline from the 5th Metatarsal Tuberosity to the Navicular bone (see diagram). Run your fingers down the lateral or outside edge of the foot until you find a slight bump, located roughly halfway between the base of the little toe and the heel. Then locate the raised Navicular bone on the medial edge of the foot (about halfway between the base of the big toe and the heel).

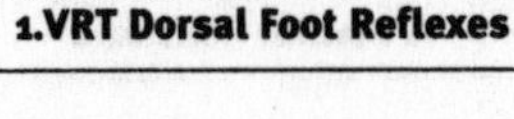

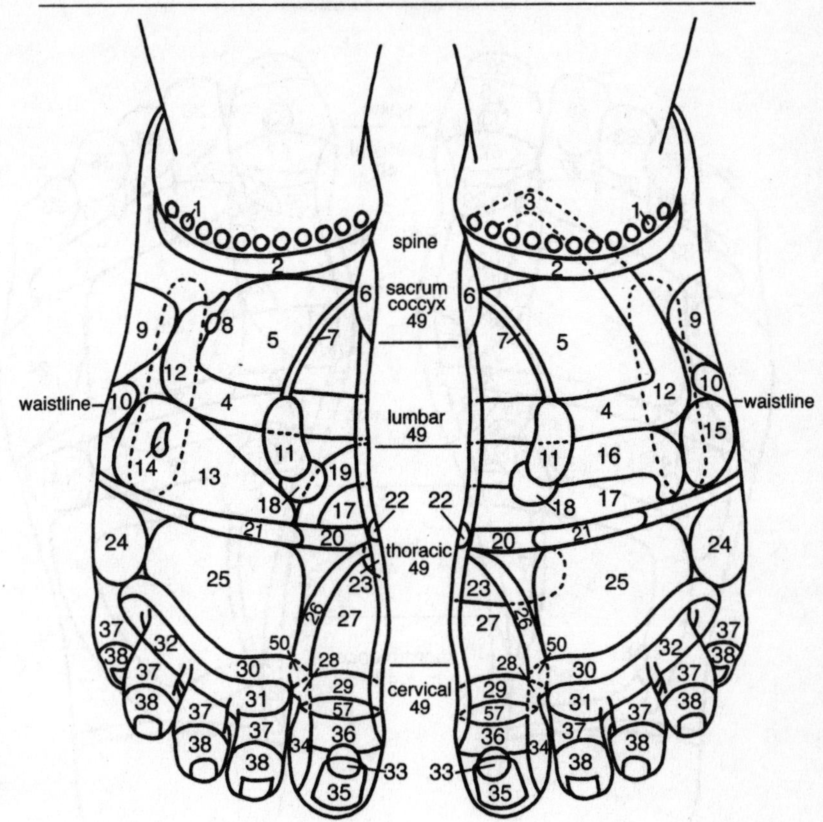

Key Master Chart for all Reflexes

1. Zonal Triggers
2. Fallopian tubes/seminal vesicles/groin/lymphatic/ vas deferens/ helper diaphragm/heart
3. Sigmoid
4. Colon
5. Small intestine
6. Bladder
7. Ureter tube
8. Appendix/ileocecal valve
9. Knee
10. Elbow
11. Kidney
12. Helper lateral digestive reflexes
13. Liver
14. Gall bladder
15. Spleen
16. Pancreas
17. Stomach
18. Adrenals
19. Duodenum
20. Diaphragm
21. Solar Plexus
22. Thymus
23. Heart
24. Shoulder
25. Chest/lung/breast
26. Trachea/oesophagus/ bronchial tubes
27. Helper Thyroid
28. Thyroid/parathyroid
29. Neck
30. Lymphatics
31. Eyes
32. Ears/Eustachian tube
33. Pituitary/Pineal/ Hypothalamus
34. Neck - side
35. Brain/skull
36. Face/teeth/ jaws/ tongue/ throat
37. Helper sinuses/teeth
38. Sinuses/brain/skull
39. Uterus/Prostate
40. Helper ovary/testes
41. Penis/vagina
42. Helper lower back/sciatic/ rectum/colon/uterus
43. Ovary/testes
44. Hip/sacro-ileac joint
45. Leg
46. Thoracic area/diaphragm
47. Hip/pelvic area
48. Helper lateral spine
49. Spine
50. Larynx/vocal cords
51. Anus/rectum
52. Armpit
53. Breastbone
54. Ribs
55. Mid/lower back
56. Sciatic nerve
57. Cerebellum/brain stem/ cranial nerves
58. Skull

2. Plantar Reflexes

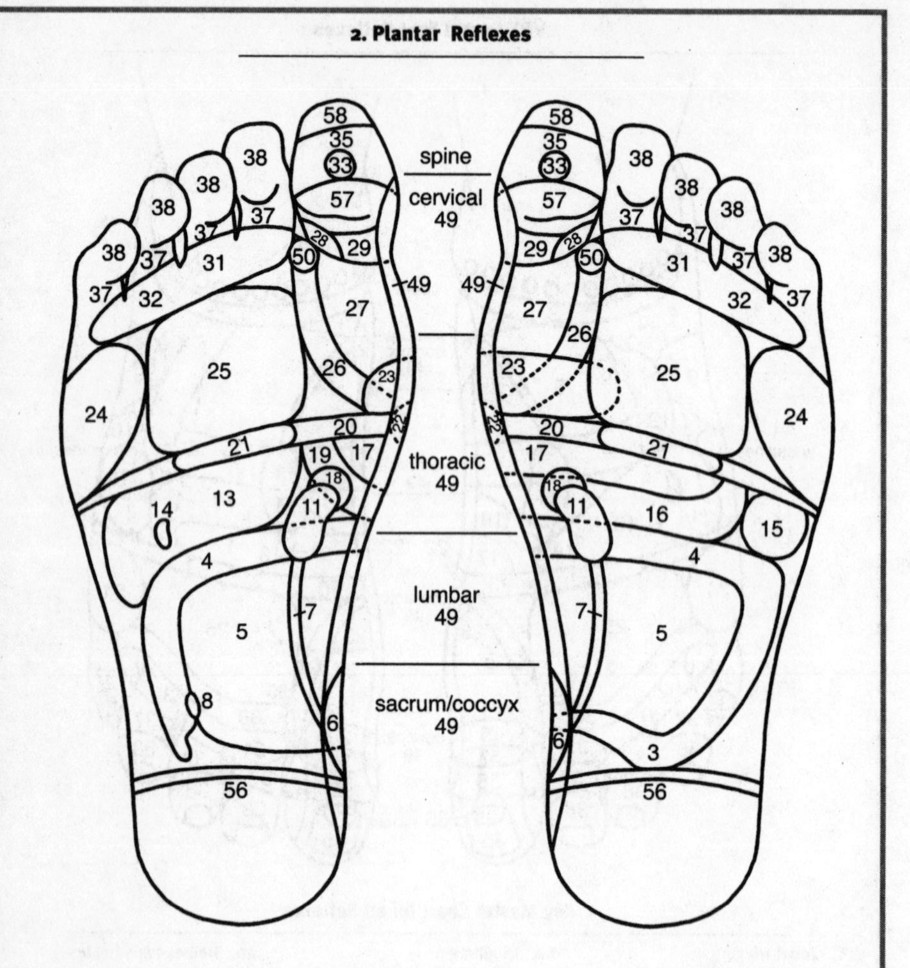

3. Sigmoid
4. Colon
5. Small intestine
6. Bladder
7. Ureter tube
8. Appendix/ileocecal valve

11. Kidney

13. Liver
14. Gall bladder
15. Spleen
16. Pancreas
17. Stomach
18. Adrenals
19. Duodenum
20. Diaphragm
21. Solar plexus
22. Thymus
23. Heart
24. Shoulder
25. Chest/lung/breast
26. Trachea/oesophagus/bronchial tubes
27. Helper thyroid
28. Thyroid/parathyroid
29. Neck

31. Eyes
32. Ears/Eustachian tube
33. Pituitary/pineal/hypothalamus

35. Brain/skull

37. Helper sinuses/teeth
38. Sinuses/brain/skull

49. Spine
50. Larynx/vocal cords

56. Sciatic nerve
57. Cerebellum/brain stem/cranial nerves
58. Skull

3. VRT Left Dorsal Foot Reflexes

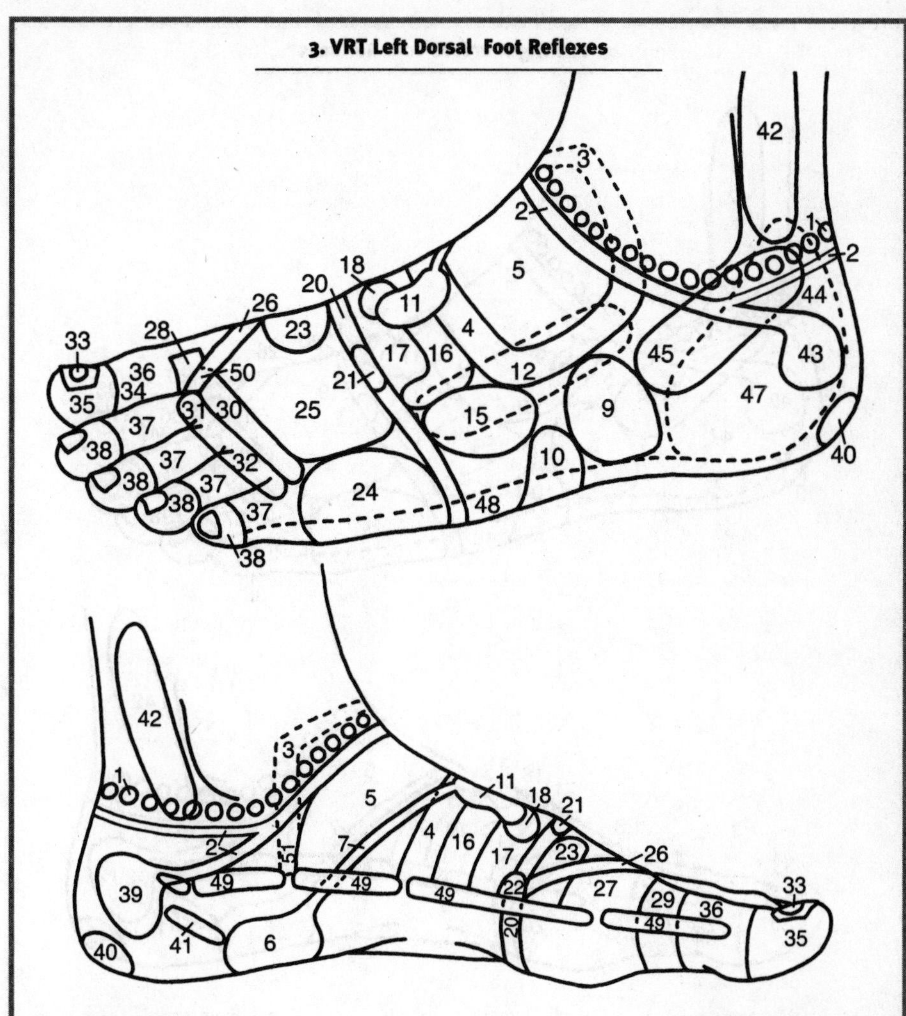

1. Zonal Triggers
2. Fallopian tubes/ seminal vesicles/vas deferens/ groin/lymphatic/helper diaphragm/heart
3. Sigmoid
4. Colon
5. Small intestine
6. Bladder
7. Ureter tube

9. Knee
10. Elbow
11. Kidney
12. Helper lateral digestive reflexes

15. Spleen
16. Pancreas
17. Stomach
18. Adrenals

20. Diaphragm
21. Solar plexus
22. Thymus
23. Heart
24. Shoulder
25. Chest/lung/breast
26. Trachea/oesophagus/ bronchial tubes
27. Helper thyroid
28. Thyroid/parathyroid
29. Neck
30. Lymphatics
31. Eyes
32. Ears/Eustachian tube
33. Pituitary/pineal/ hypothalamus
34. Neck – side
35. Brain/skull
36. Face/teeth/ jaws/ tongue/ throat
37. Helper sinuses/teeth
38. Sinuses/brain/skull
39. Uterus/prostate
40. Helper ovary/testes
41. Penis/vagina
42. Helper lower back/sciatic/ rectum/colon/uterus
43. Ovary/testes
44. Hip/sacro-ileac joint
45. Leg

47. Hip/pelvic area
48. Helper lateral spine
49. Spine
50. Larynx/vocal cords

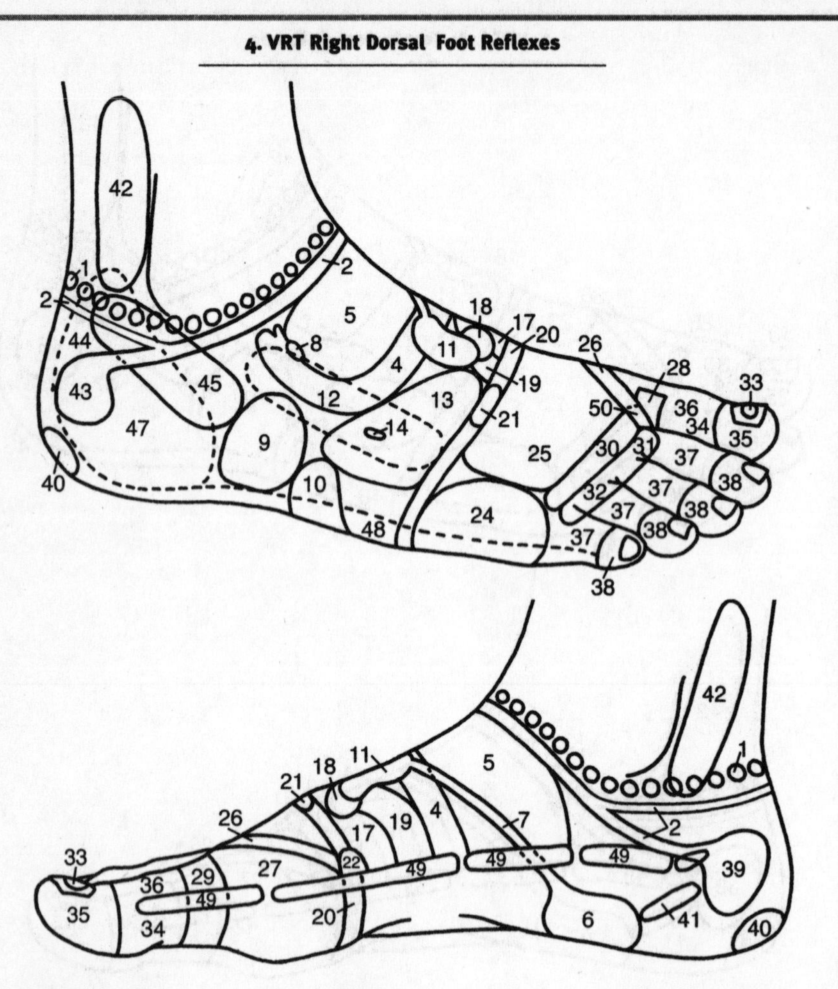

4. VRT Right Dorsal Foot Reflexes

1. Zonal Triggers
2. Fallopian tubes/ seminal vesicles/ vas deferens/ groin/lymphatic/helper diaphragm/heart

4. Colon
5. Small intestine
6. Bladder
7. Ureter tube
8. Appendix/ileocecal valve
9. Knee
10. Elbow
11. Kidney
12. Helper lateral digestive reflexes
13. Liver
14. Gall bladder

17. Stomach
18. Adrenals
19. Duodenum
20. Diaphragm
21. Solar plexus
22. Thymus

24. Shoulder
25. Chest/lung/breast
26. Trachea/ oesophagus/bronchial tubes
27. Helper thyroid
28. Thyroid/parathyroid
29. Neck
30. Lymphatics
31. Eyes
32. Ears/Eustachian tube
33. Pituitary/pineal/ hypothalamus
34. Neck – side
35. Brain/skull
36. Face/teeth/ jaws/ tongue/ throat
37. Helper sinuses/teeth
38. Sinuses/brain/skull
39. Uterus/prostate
40. Helper ovary/testes
41. Penis/vagina
42. Helper lower back/sciatic/ rectum/colon/uterus
43. Ovary/testes
44. Hip/sacro-ileac joint
45. Leg

47. Hip/pelvic area
48. Helper lateral spine
49. Spine
50. Larynx/vocal cords

5. VRT Thoracic Calf Reflexes

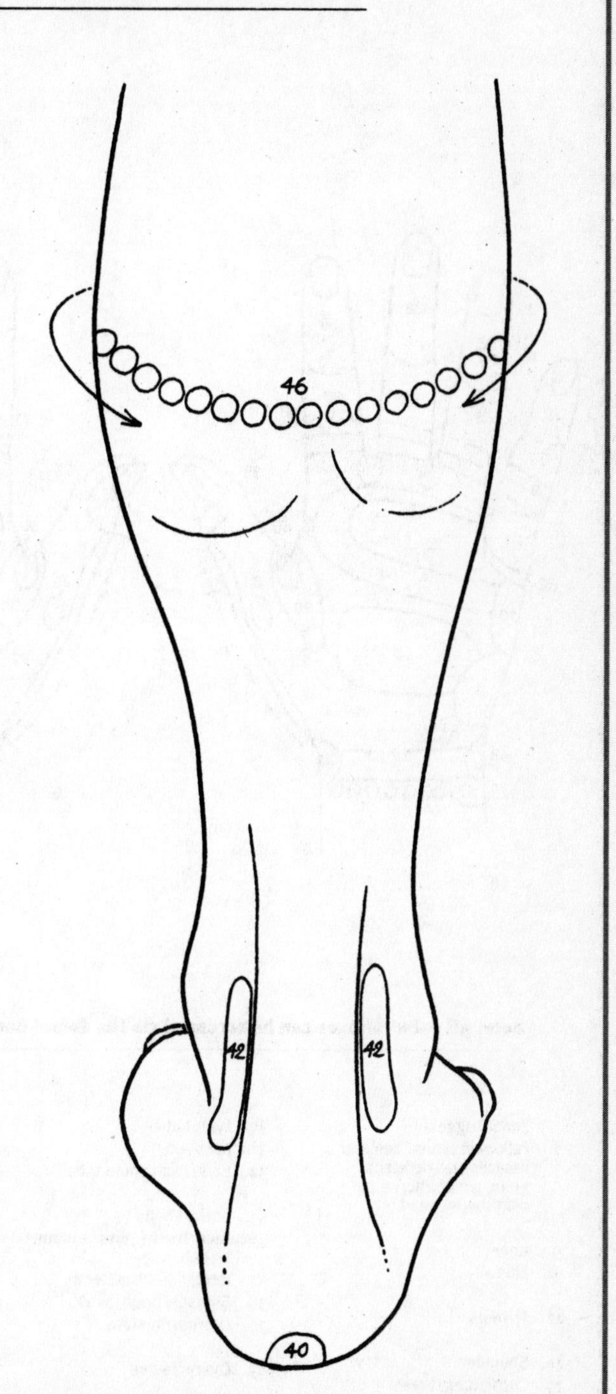

40. Helper ovary/testes

42. Helper lower back/sciatic/ rectum/colon/uterus

46. Thoracic area/diaphragm

6. VRT Dorsal Hand Reflexes

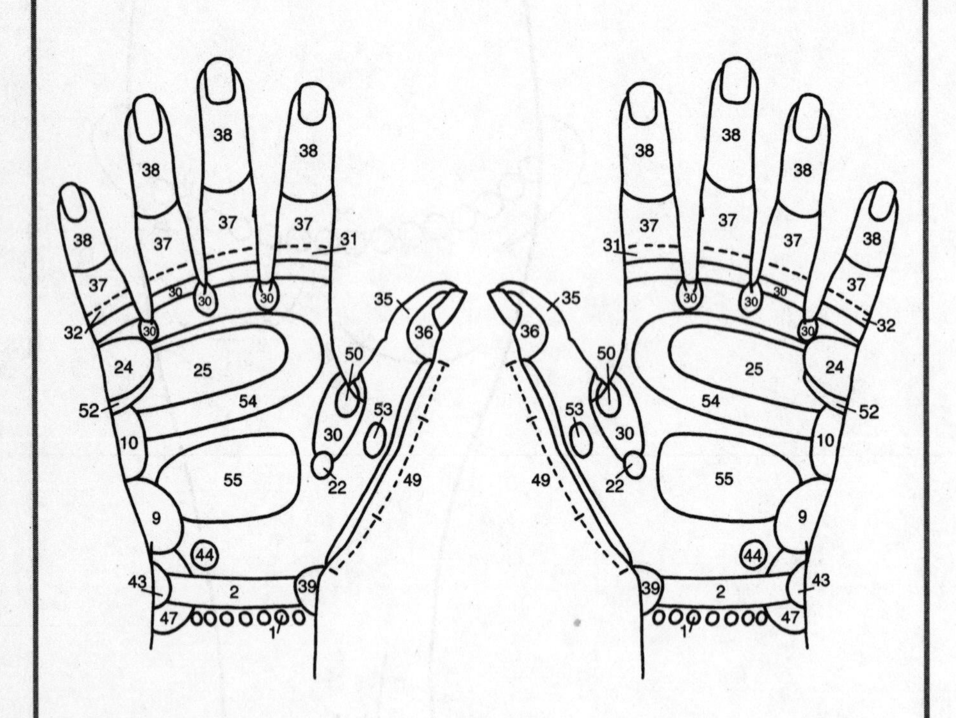

Note: All palm reflexes can be accessed via the dorsal hand when weight-bearing.

1. Zonal Triggers
2. Fallopian tubes/ seminal vesicles/vas deferens/ groin/lymphatic/helper diaphragm/heart
9. Knee
10. Elbow
22. Thymus
24. Shoulder
25. Chest/lung/breast
30. Lymphatics
31. Eyes
32. Ears/Eustachian tube
35. Brain/skull
36. Face/teeth/ jaws/ tongue/ throat
37. Helper sinuses/teeth
38. Sinuses/brain/skull
39. Uterus/prostate
43. Ovary/testes
44. Hip/sacro-ileac joint
47. Hip/pelvic area
49. Spine
50. Larynx/vocal cords
52. Armpit
53. Breastbone
54. Ribs
55. Mid/lower back

7. VRT Palm Reflexes

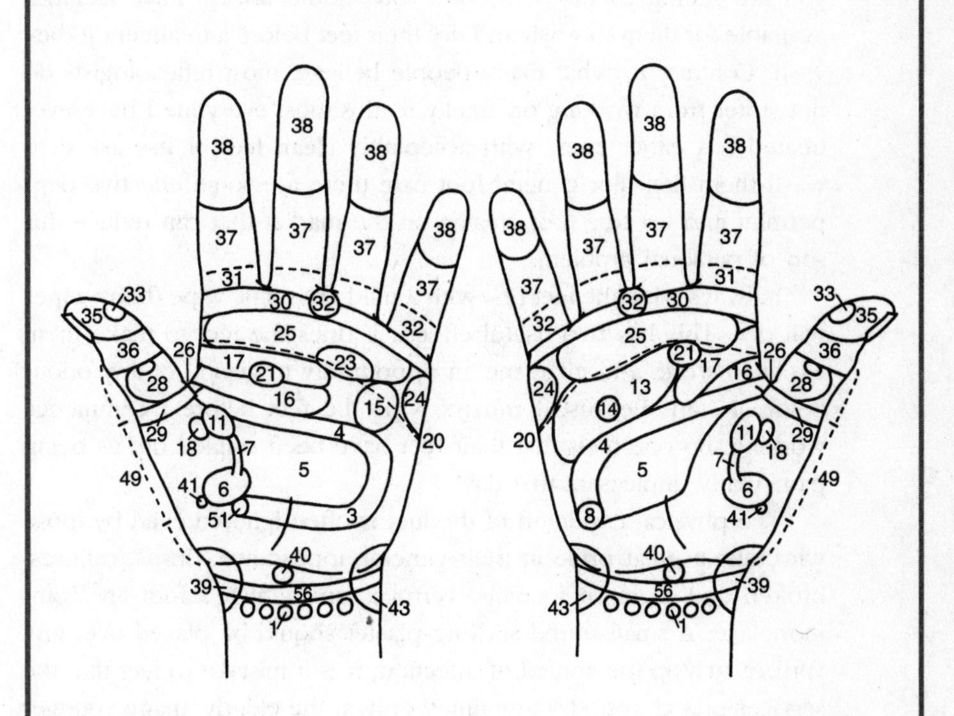

1. Zonal Triggers
3. Sigmoid
4. Colon
5. Small intestine
6. Bladder
7. Ureter tube
8. Appendix/ileocecal valve
11. Kidney
13. Liver
14. Gall bladder
15. Spleen
16. Pancreas
17. Stomach
18. Adrenals
20. Diaphragm
21. Solar Plexus
23. Heart
24. Shoulder
25. Chest/lung/breast
26. Trachea/oesophagus/ bronchial tubes
28. Thyroid/parathyroid
29. Neck
30. Lymphatics
31. Eyes
32. Ears/Eustachian tube
33. Pituitary/pineal/ hypothalamus
35. Brain/skull
36. Face/teeth/ jaws/ tongue/ throat
37. Helper sinuses/teeth
38. Sinuses/brain/skull
39. Uterus/prostate
40. Helper ovary/testes
41. Penis/vagina
43. Ovary/testes
49. Spine
51. Anus/rectum
56. Sciatic nerve

Preparing the feet for VRT and reflexology

Condition of the feet

It helps if, before treatment, every client has prepared their feet by making sure that they are clean and the toenails are cut short. Whether you are seeing clients or friends you should always have facilities available for them to wash and dry their feet before a treatment if they wish. Contrary to what many people believe, most reflexologists do not suffer from working on smelly feet! Almost everyone I have ever treated has either come with acceptably clean feet or has asked to wash them first. For general foot care there are some effective peppermint and tea tree foot creams on the market that can reduce this sort of personal problem.

I always wipe the feet first with a mild antiseptic wipe (baby wipes will do). This has two useful effects: it dries the feet to make them easier to work, and gives me an opportunity to get rid of any odour before I start. Because I *always* wipe the feet before I commence working, no one feels that their feet have been singled out as being particularly unpleasant that day!

The physical condition of the feet is often ignored even by those who take a great pride in their general appearance. Corns, calluses, broken and ingrown toenails, verrucas and athlete's foot are commonplace. A small round sticking plaster should be placed over any verruca to stop the spread of infection. It is a mistake to feel that the services of a chiropodist are aimed only at the elderly: many younger people could benefit from periodical treatment to prevent minor problems becoming entrenched. Self-help includes rubbing dry skin gently with a pumice during the daily bath or shower. For hard skin on the toes and heel, massage the feet with calendula oil each night for a week or so and the skin will often soften like magic. Unromantic as it sounds, you should then put on a pair of old socks so that the oil does not stain your sheets!

Athlete's foot can spread all over the feet and, of course, on to other people's feet as well via swimming pools and changing rooms. Tea tree oil preparations can help cure this highly infectious condition and help to keep it at bay. Alternatively, consult your doctor.

As long as the feet are clean, whatever their condition, they can be worked on confidently and easily. Many potential clients, friends and family want to experience reflexology and VRT but are too embarrassed and suggest waiting for a treatment until they have had their feet seen to! Assure them that their feet are not a problem for *you*, and that the sooner they receive reflexology the sooner their general health will improve. Women in their sixties are particularly apologetic about their bunions, corns and calluses as they were fashion victims of the 1950s' winklepicker shoes. Common areas of hard skin are often found on the heels and toes, due to ill-fitting shoes. If a foot has a open wound, is sore or has a problem varicose vein, simply work the corresponding hand instead.

It has never been proved, but there are many reports of headaches ceasing after having an ingrown toenail removed. This seems to suggest that, in some cases, there may be undue pressure on the head/brain reflexes which aggravate the head itself.

Many reflexologists have also observed that certain parts of the foot are subtly different in colour or texture, blotchy, or may be callused or covered in dry skin. This sometimes appears to be a reflection of a malfunction in the reflexes of the foot which are situated in the same area. For example, people with respiratory problems often find that the ball of the foot (lung/bronchial area) has hard, dry skin. Over a period of reflexology sessions the thickened skin softens and clears and becomes naturally smoother as the client's general health improves.

Finally, Vertical Reflex Therapy is even less threatening than reflexology to those who apologise profusely for the state of their feet. They simply stand for a few minutes in a position where a large percentage of their feet is hidden!

Relaxing the feet

Now for some standard relaxation techniques. If you intend to only practise VRT you will not need to learn these techniques, as the people you treat will not need to sit or lie down. However, I would encourage everyone to use relaxation techniques and Diaphragm Rocking (see Chapter 7) as often as possible, as they consolidate the VRT and help the body make extra corrections.

Requirements for all conventional reflexology and VRT treatments

Although reflexologists can use their hands on pairs of feet anywhere, it is useful to be equipped, or make use of, the following:

- Short, neatly cut fingernails and clean hands.
- Clean towel on which to stand.
- Mild antiseptic or baby wipes.
- Tissues to pat the feet dry.
- Non-oily cream or specialist foot cream – an optional but very useful item when working into the reflexes on the foot. A minute amount of cream should be used, to give light lubrication only.
- Corn starch – if you wish to work on a very dry foot use corn starch (cornflour).
- A glass of water – reflexology, and especially VRT, stimulate the body to make positive changes, including the release and excretion of harmful toxins. Water can help flush these out quickly, so all clients should be encouraged to drink more water especially on the day of treatment. This helps prevent the possibility of a slight headache caused by a temporary rise of toxins in the bloodstream.
- Ideally you should treat people in a quiet, warm room where you cannot be disturbed and the telephone can be ignored. Remember that this is their dedicated time, whether five minutes or a full hour.

Specific requirements for VRT

- Optional non-oily foot cream.
- Optional cushion to kneel on.
- Upright chair or table for support.

Specific requirements for conventional reflexology

- A therapist's padded couch or a reclining chair (you can improvise by using a bed or an easy chair with a cushion on a stool to rest the feet – but make sure you do not sit at an uncomfortable angle).

- A swivel office-type chair so that you can move freely to work the feet from different angles.
- A reflexologist's portable tilting stool, such as the Porta-ped brand (see p. 185), on which to place the feet when the client is in a chair – essential for home visits.

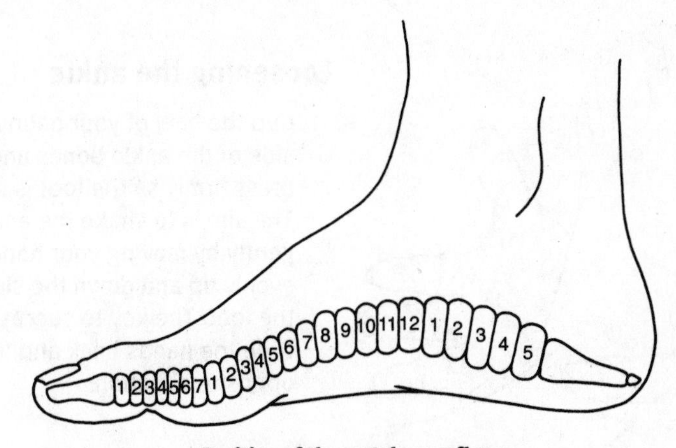

Position of the vertebrae reflexes

Case study

When a young woman complained of inexplicable headaches and tired eyes I worked her eye reflexes thoroughly at the base of all her toes and then moved on to the neck reflexes on her big toe to ease the headaches. I did some relaxation techniques to loosen up the spine generally, then returned to her toes at the end. This time the eye reflex under the second toe was very tender, and within a minute her eye had begun to stream. Later she saw an optician, who diagnosed a blocked tear duct. It was only after I had stimulated the neck reflexes and returned to a particular part of the eye that the body responded and the blocked tear duct began to clear. Her body obviously needed to relax first before energy could be directed to help the eye.

Relaxation techniques

First touch the feet of the person you are treating and make positive contact by firmly holding them both. It is helpful to grasp each heel firmly and pull them a little towards you to stretch the legs a fraction. When you relax or work the feet it makes no difference whether you begin with the left or right foot.

The following relaxation techniques are to be used when a person is lying down. They can be introduced at the beginning of conventional reflexology treatments, and are also used in conjunction with Complete VRT when the person lies back briefly in between short VRT treatments and experiences reflexology and Diaphragm Rocking.

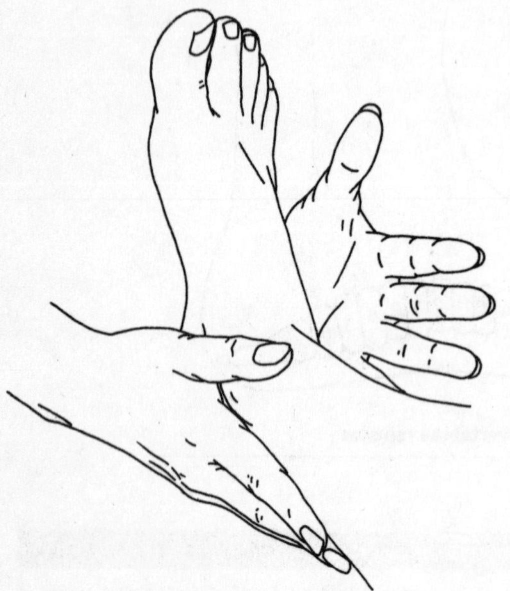

Loosening the ankle

Cup the heel of your palms either side of the ankle bones and press firmly so the foot is secure. The aim is to shake the ankle gently by moving your hands evenly up and down the sides of the foot. The key to success is to slide the hands back and forth in opposite directions.

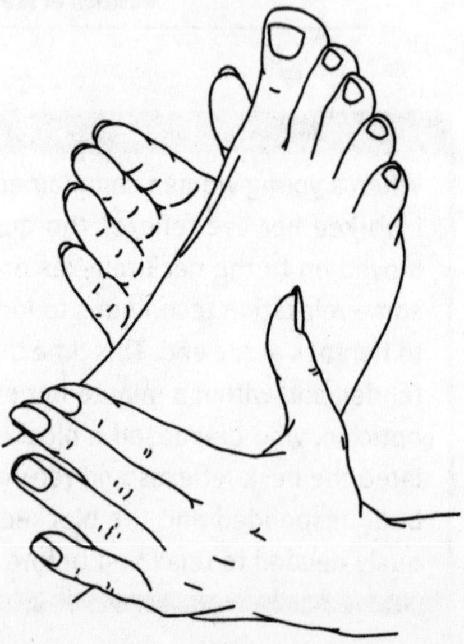

As the right hand moves forward the left hand is sliding backwards a little, and then the movement is reversed. Once you are confident in the movement allow your fingers and upper hand to become more flexible so that they gently slap the sides of the feet as you work. Repeat on the other foot.

Twisting the spinal reflexes

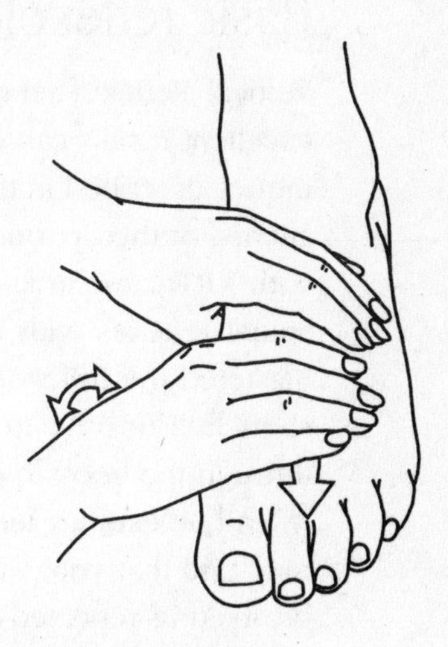

Turn the foot so that it naturally splays outwards and place both hands, side by side, over the top of the foot with your fingers pointing to the outside edge of the foot. Let your two thumbs touch the sole of the foot and press the webbing of your thumb firmly against the spinal reflexes on the inside edge of the foot. Do not move the hand closest to the ankles but simply use it to grip the foot firmly. The other hand grips and turns the foot in a rotating movement backwards and forwards. Do not twist the foot too far or it will be a painful instead of a pleasant stretching sensation. Rock the part of the foot nearest the toes two or three times, then slide both hands about 2 cm towards the toes and repeat the movements. Continue up the foot until the edge of your hand (the little finger) covers the toes. Repeat on the other foot.

Whole body brush

Place your hands over the feet with your fingertips touching the ankle band and pointing towards the legs. Press your eight fingers gently but firmly on the skin and simultaneously move both hands towards you in tiny, slightly jerky little bites. The whole movement should flow from the ankle to the toes, but the client should be aware of pressure as your fingers move across the top of their foot. The movements are made three times on each foot by returning to the ankles. The first pass along the feet should be firm and stimulating, but the second should be lighter and allow your fingers to slide more. The third time you work over the foot it should be a gentle brushing soothing movement with your fingertips. Repeat on the other foot.

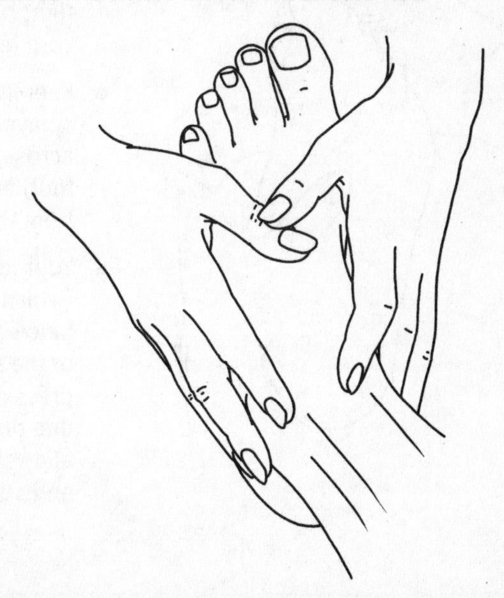

Basic reflexology techniques

Vertical Reflex Therapy in its basic form is very simple to use, and excellent results can be obtained by using the small selection of techniques described in this chapter. Many reflexologists have taught their clients, or their partners, the basic VRT skills. Some of my best results with VRT came in its earliest days when I just pressed the ankles and spinal reflexes with my index finger or knuckle. So once you have mastered the following techniques you will be equipped to give the short holistic VRT treatment. Then you have the choice to move on through the book to discover more techniques as your skills develop.

All reflexology techniques take time to perfect. As you practise you may find that your fingers and thumbs become quite stiff, as you will be making repeated movements with some tiny, little used muscles and joints. Be careful not to overwork them in the early days, and make sure when you approach the feet that your hands are always working at the most comfortable angle with the least strain. In fact, observe how you use your whole body so that you do not place undue stress upon it.

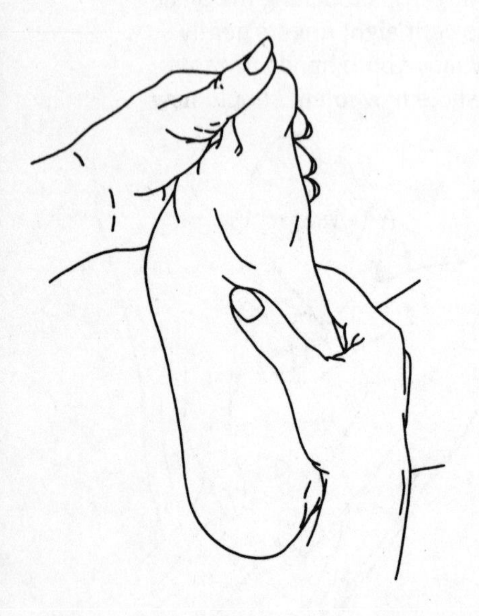

Holding the foot

- Hold the right foot with your left hand and use your right hand to work the reflexes. Then hold the left foot with your right hand and the working hand will be your left.
- Keeping the foot upright and slightly splayed outwards, place your hand across the metatarsals (the top of the foot) and the toes – you will be gripping from the outer side of the foot.
- Your left thumb and thenar muscle (which is the part of the palm directly below the thumb) will cover the top part of the sole with the tip of the thumb pressing on the tip of the big toe. This is one of the basic reflexology holds that allows you to work the sole of the foot and support it at the same time.

Thumb pressure walking

Most reflexology techniques are best practised on your own hands and arms first to feel the pressure and sensation they produce. The thumb is used extensively in reflexology – but it is usually the outer side that is used, sometimes the tip and certainly not the nail.

- Place your left hand palm down on a table and place your right thumb firmly on to the top of your hand pressing with the tip or edge of your thumb. It is important to bend your thumb about 45 degrees at the first joint, the one nearest the nail. If the thumb is straight, or bent on the second joint, it will become strained and will not be at the correct angle to work the reflexes.
- Now inch the thumb along in tiny movements as if you are pressing on a series of pinpoints. Try the same movements on your other hand, and this time press firmly into your skin so that you are aware of different sensations as you work. This is often referred to as the 'caterpillar walking' technique.
- Become aware of the fleshy and bony parts of your hands, of rough skin, of whether the hand feels warm or cool, and see if the pressure of your thumb causes any parts of your hand to feel tender.

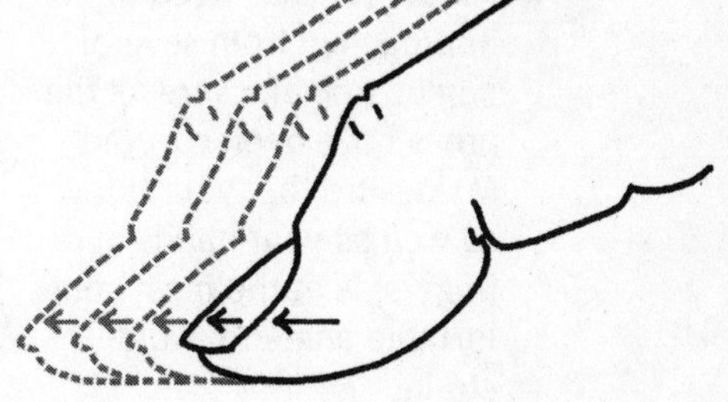

Your aim is to develop a firm, even pressure and a sensitivity to changes in the feel of the hands and feet which could indicate that a particular reflex needs stimulating. Do not expect to feel anything much at first, though you can still achieve results simply by pressing the right reflexes as shown in the charts. Some reflexologists are very successful because they work the feet thoroughly and cover all the reflexes, but they rarely get much information back from the feet. Other practitioners work extremely intuitively on the feet and may be able to tell that a part of the body is sore, inflamed or painful just by the feel of the reflexes. Both approaches are acceptable. More to the point, both methods achieve results. The side of your thumb is extremely versatile in reaching all parts of the foot. Remember to work slowly and rhythmically as you creep your thumb across the foot or hands.

If you want to practise reflexology techniques, I recommend that you buy a cheap latex hand and foot from a joke shop! Some will be unsuitable and grotesque, but many are from moulds taken from a human hand or foot. My own demonstration foot is excellent and came from a joke shop in South Carolina. However, before using it as a teaching aid I had to carefully scrape off a large amount of fake blood from the ankle!

Finger pressure walking

The same principles and techniques apply to fingers and thumbs when the reflexes are worked.

- Use the middle to outer edge of the index or forefinger and bend the first joint only at an angle of 45 degrees as it works across the foot. If you keep your finger completely straight or bent at the other joints, not only will it put more strain on your fingers but you will not be able to locate the reflexes so accurately.
- Tender reflexes need to be approached from several angles to make sure all the areas have been covered. Make sure that your body, as well as your hands and fingers, is at the most comfortable angle to avoid strain.

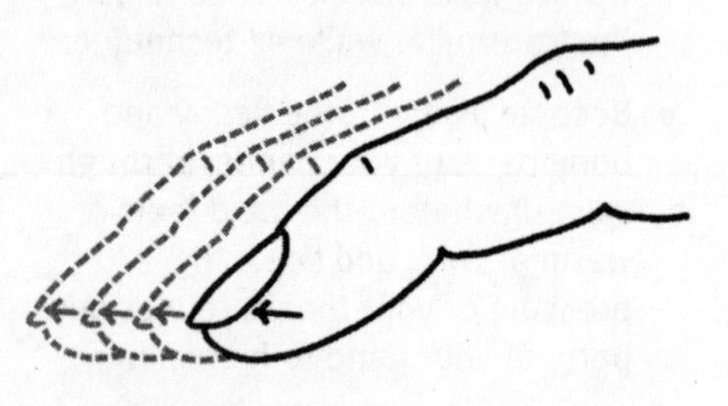

Some VRT techniques in Chapter 5 use three or four fingers, and the emphasis is on the fingertips pressing and brushing the skin. Again, for comfort and greatest effect the first joint of the finger should be the only one that is bent. If the finger is straight, the nails can dig in and cause pain. Sometimes a reflex can feel sore, tender or gritty to the touch – in reflexology this is a positive sensation which is known as a good hurt! It is suggested that these tiny crystal deposits felt in the feet are connected to a particular reflex and are a reflection of an imbalance in the body. The side of the finger can work into these points from different angles and often achieves a three-fold effect of dispersing the granulation, easing the tenderness in the reflex and improving the condition in the corresponding part of the body.

The use of knuckles in reflexology

Some reflexologists have developed many new techniques by using their knuckles as well as their fingers and thumbs. There is a surprising degree of sensitivity in the side of the knuckle, especially when working the spine, hip, pelvic and knee reflexes around the sides of the ankles.

My former tutor, Anthony Porter of ART (Advanced Reflexology Training), has pioneered and developed many new techniques and treatments that incorporate the use of knuckles and a tiny amount of foot cream. I was very interested in the potential use of ART techniques combined with VRT because it enabled me to access many of the standing reflexes easily. It helped me to work more effectively and stopped me straining my fingers and thumbs all the time. Professional reflexologists are at risk from repetitive strain injuries, and the ART techniques help to spread the load so that the conventionally used finger and thumb joints are given a partial rest.

To a few reflexologists the use of cream and knuckles is an anathema as their training expressly forbids it. I respect their professional view, and avoidance of this method will not impede their results with VRT. For all willing to experiment, the following instructions supply enough information to allow them to work the standing or relaxed foot in a very effective and powerful way.

Cream and knuckles

Wipe the feet with an antiseptic wipe and work on them at first without cream. Reflexology is not a foot massage, and you only require a tiny amount of cream to help you work into a reflex. The cream should be non-oily – ordinary hand cream can be used if you do not have any proprietary foot cream. As you work particular reflexes, take a tiny speck of cream and work it into the reflexes in a rotating movement with your fingertip. Do not under any circumstances cover the foot in cream and try to slip and slide your way through an inadequate treatment!

This one technique will enable you to work the relaxed feet in a specific and powerful way, and it is incredibly effective on the standing foot. Orthopaedic problems sometimes respond almost instantly when a knuckle gently works the hip, knee and pelvic reflexes around the ankle bones.

Practise using the knuckle

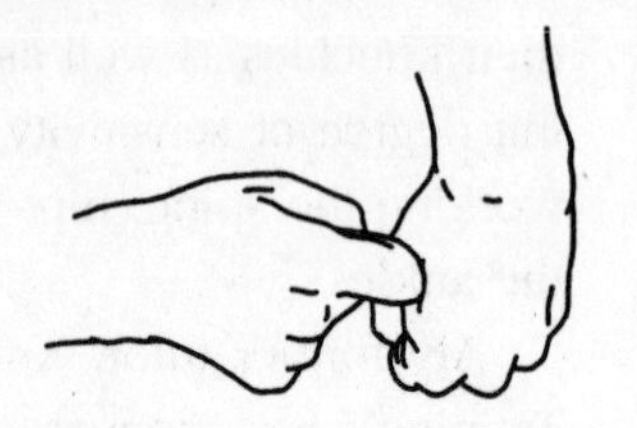

- Bend all your fingers at the second joint to form a knuckle.
- Tuck your thumb loosely under your fingers or leave it naturally outstretched if it suits you better as you work.
- Now slightly raise the knuckle of your index finger and practise on your other hand by pressing and twisting it into your hand.
- You will be aware of a surprisingly precise area of contact, and if you incline your knuckle slightly to the outer side you will be able to locate reflexes even more accurately.

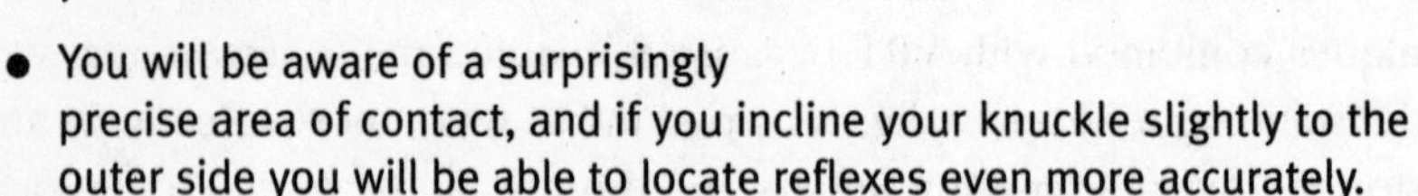

Method using the tip of the knuckle

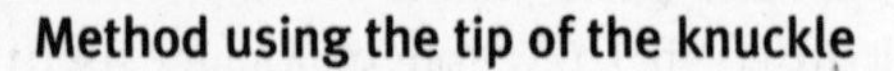

- Press the reflex with your knuckle in the same way that you would use your finger, and rock your hands slightly backwards and forwards from the wrist.
- Now work the foot so that you feel the knuckle stretch the surface as it slides up and down the foot for about 2 cm.
- Return to the same point and repeat the pressing and sliding motion two or three times.
- Use just enough lubrication to allow the knuckle to slide slowly back and forward over the reflexes.

Method using the side of the knuckle

- Using the same standard knuckle position on each hand, point your two index finger knuckles at the hip/pelvic reflexes on either side of the ankle on the left or right foot.

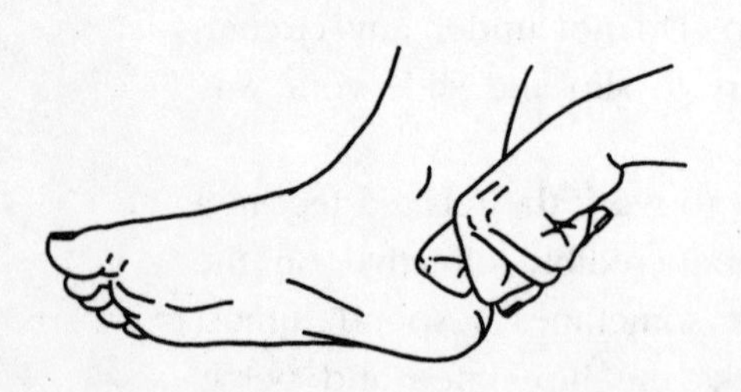

- Using the inner side of your knuckles, rotate both fists at once on the reflexes directly under the ankle.
- Add a tiny amount of cream, and slide and press the knuckles simultaneously in a circular movement.
- This is a powerful conventional technique used on the foot when lying down and an extremely effective VRT technique used on the standing foot, for a maximum of 30 seconds per foot.

Case study

Sarah was a newly qualified reflexologist when she attended one of my VRT courses. I demonstrated on her feet as she was suffering from a trapped nerve running from her shoulder to her fingers. Although it did not prevent her treating clients, the shoulder was so painful that she was considering giving up her day job. At the end of the workshop she told the group that the pain in her arm had nearly disappeared after only a few minutes of VRT. Within days it had gone completely and did not return, and she was able to resume driving. She subsequently used VRT to 'brilliant effect' on a client with a whiplash injury.

Practice is essential when working with your hands in an unfamiliar way, but you will soon become accustomed to using your knuckles. Reflexologists who trained in the ART techniques have told me that they feel they gain extra digits once the use of knuckles is introduced.

Advantages of VRT to the therapist

Reflexology is a particularly non-active and restrictive therapy from a manual point of view, as reflexologists sit still and just move their hands, fingers and thumbs. Vertical Reflex Therapy offers them much more flexibility of movement and most VRT techniques can be used conventionally as well. This allows the therapist to stand and move about to hold the hands and feet if the person is lying down. All the VRT techniques are applied when the therapist is kneeling or sitting on the floor, which allows him or her a brief stretch at the start and end of treatments. Anyone who regularly practises VRT may well become slightly more active and energetic as he or she works, due to the different usage of knuckles, fingers and even palms.

With the basics of reflexology covered, you are now ready to move on to learning how to give a Basic VRT treatment in Chapter 5.

Key points to remember

- Familiarise yourself with the foot charts before you begin treating anyone.
- Have a regular professional reflexology treatment yourself, whether or not you are a reflexologist.
- Basic VRT can be used as an effective five-minute treatment in its own right.
- Complete VRT is a comprehensive twenty-minute treatment that comprises a short reflexology treatment with a few minutes of VRT either side.
- VRT can be added at the beginning and/or end of all conventional reflexology treatments.
- Relaxation techniques should be included with five-minute Basic VRT whenever possible.
- All VRT techniques can be used repeatedly on the feet when in a reclining position, as they are helpful but much less powerful.
- Experiment with knuckles and new techniques so that you make less repetitive movements with your fingers.
- Take care of your feet and pamper them. Consider having a treatment from a chiropodist – whatever your age!

Step-by-step instructions for Basic VRT

IF USED AS PART OF TRADITIONAL REFLEXOLOGY VRT SHOULD NORMALLY NOT take more than about eight minutes in total. That means a maximum of five minutes at the start and another two to three minutes at the conclusion of a treatment. If used in isolation it should take about five minutes from start to finish.

The following VRT treatment is short and each session should take a maximum of four to five minutes. It may take you longer in the early practice stages, but while learning be careful not to overwork any particular reflexes – work any part of the foot for a few seconds only and move on.

Preparation

- Talk to the client or partner and ascertain if there are any problems that may affect the use of VRT, such as giddiness, varicose veins or an inability to stand for any length of time. Even if you are treating a friend or family member it is best to check that there are no problems of which you may not be aware.
- If you are dealing with an orthopaedic condition, test the range of mobility before and after the session. This not only helps you to access the problem but may well prove an excellent demonstration of the power of VRT.
- Read the list of requirements on p. 80 and supply yourself with what you need.

'What does "overworking the reflexes" mean?'

It means too much stimulation has been placed on a reflex during a treatment, and the body has responded with a headache, feelings of nausea or increased pain. In extreme cases it can bring about a healing crisis – the body over-reacts before it gets better, and tries to throw off all the accumulated toxins too quickly.

Case study

Margaret, aged sixty, was diagnosed with arthritis and osteoporosis and suffered pain and stiffness in the left hip, groin and knee. She had suffered a fall several months before, but her prescribed painkillers made her feel tired and had ceased to alleviate the extreme discomfort which kept her awake at night. Her work involved climbing many stairs and she gained only temporary relief from hydrotherapy treatments. When she received five minutes of Basic VRT before she started work, her knee instantly became less painful. She then had two more minutes on the pelvic, spinal and knee reflexes before she left. By the next day the pain had decreased enough for her to leave off the painkillers for good. Within a week she had more energy, more mobility in her hip and less knee and groin pain. Top-ups of a few minutes of VRT twice a week, and her own daily self-help treatments, keep her fairly agile and relatively pain-free.

Position and posture

The correct VRT position

Always ensure that the person treated is standing straight but relaxed, knees slightly bent, and is able to steady themselves by holding on to a table or chair. *Never* allow them to stand on a stool or chair, however much more convenient it is for you, as they could easily lose their balance and fall. Some people suggest standing on a second or third stair, holding on to the banisters, while they have their feet worked by someone kneeling on the floor at the bottom. I would not advise this position as people can feel quite light-headed during VRT and could fall forward, hurting themselves and you. If you are a practising therapist you will be insured; if you are just treating friends you may not be. Either way, such an unpleasant outcome is not worth the risk under any circumstances.

If the reflexologist has a problem herself and cannot kneel or sit, the client can stand and put one foot at a time on a chair, leaning forward slightly to increase the pressure as the foot is worked. The therapist can then sit on an adjacent chair, or use a small stool.

'Should VRT and reflexology hurt?'

Both therapies are basically relaxing and pleasant experiences, but a tender reflex will often cause a momentary feeling of discomfort or pain. At this point the reflexologist will immediately work it more lightly. But there should never be any lasting hurt or pain.

The correct posture for the practitioner

The practitioner must be prepared to move around on their knees or backside for a few minutes! Have a cushion available to kneel on if necessary. Another alternative is to have a small wooden sloping 'prayer stool' to sit on. These are only a few centimetres from the ground and you slip your legs underneath the seat. Remember to move your body as well as your hands. Bad posture caused by twisting instead of moving can cause unnecessary pressure on the back, wrists and shoulders. Keep your arms as close to the floor as possible to avoid straining them downwards at an angle. If the client is able to move freely, does not get giddy and has something to hold on to, ask them to move round until they are in the correct position for a particular movement. This is also helpful if you are working in a confined space.

'So what is the difference between a healing crisis and side-effects?'

A healing crisis, is stronger than side-effects, which are also very short-lived. Side-effects, as the body is stimulated to dispose of toxins, can include minor muzziness, thirst, mild skin outbreaks or slightly increased output of urine or faeces. VRT can sometimes cause an increase in pain for a few hours, especially when dealing with mobility problems, before recovery takes place. Drinking plenty of water will help minimise any side-effects. In a healing crisis you may have to evacuate your bowels several times a day, or pass large quantities of cloudy urine, and you may feel considerable pain. While not pleasant, both side-effects and the symptoms of a healing crisis will quickly pass, and should be welcomed as a sign that the body is healing itself.

The importance of alternating the feet

It is essential that the feet are treated alternately at every stage because the person needs to be kept in balance by constantly stimulating the reflexes on both sides of the body. If you fail to do so, the other side of the body can feel very lop-sided and limp. So do not treat one foot completely before you work the second. The only exception is when you are using self-help techniques (see Chapter 9), when the body is working within your own energy field and can cope with one foot at a time being worked.

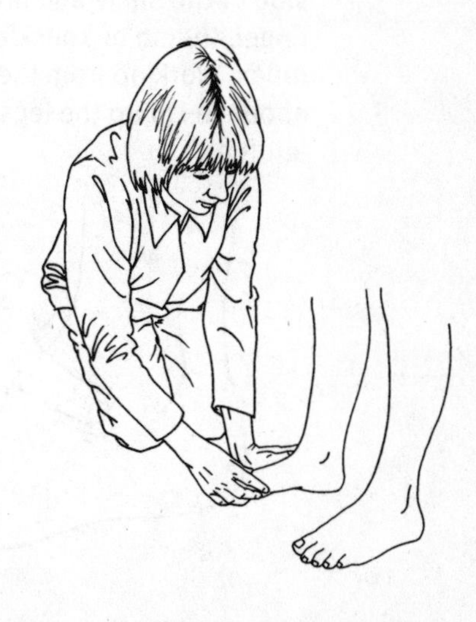

Basic method for Vertical Reflex Therapy

For continuity in the instructions we will always start with the right foot. Consult the main foot charts in Chapter 4 when necessary.

Ankles first

Very important! Always start with the ankle reflexes first. These points open up the body to a deeper healing response.

Ankle reflexes – to stimulate the immune system

Kneel down and face the client's feet, or ask them to turn their back to you and you can work the ankles from behind. Experiment to discover which is easier for you. Use the knuckles or fingers of both hands simultaneously on the right foot, and work into the hip, pelvic and sciatic reflexes on both sides of the ankle. Brush your thumb across the top of the ankle (groin/fallopian tube/seminal vesicle/*vas deferens* reflexes), noting any particularly painful point. You will return to this area later in more detail when using Synergistic Reflexology.

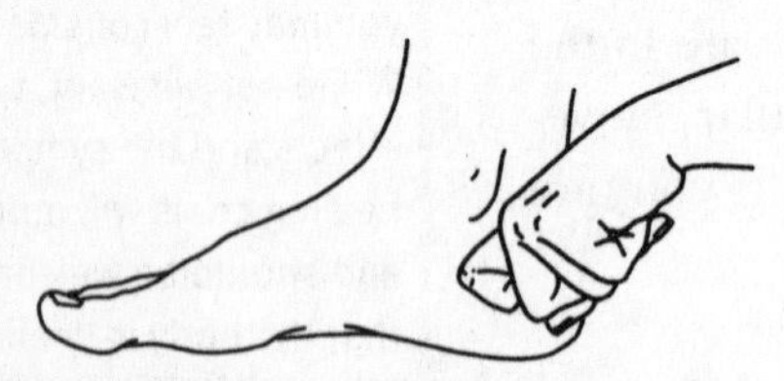

Work the reproductive reflexes below each side of the ankle and press and rotate your finger, thumb or knuckle over the bladder reflex. Work up from the ankle bones to about 10 cm up the legs. Repeat on the left foot.

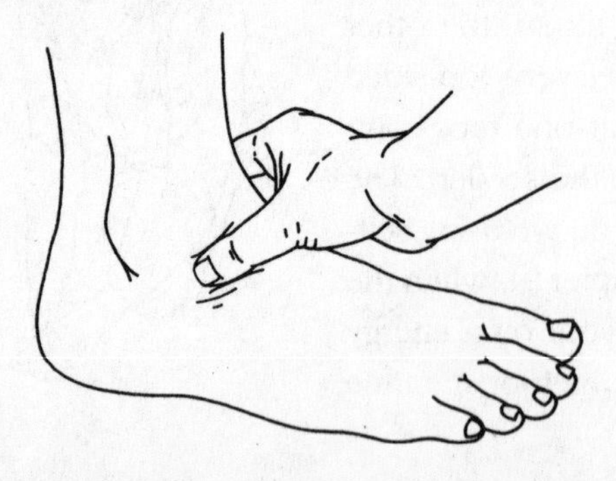

Reminder: key steps

- **Work under and over the ankle bones simultaneously on both sides of the foot.**
- **Slide your thumb backwards and forwards across the ankle 'bracelet'.**
- **Stimulate the bladder and reproductive reflexes.**
- **Work your fingers simultaneously up either side of the ankles – this stimulates the sciatic reflexes and locates helper colon reflexes.**
- **Repeat on the other foot.**

The next three moves; the lumbar spine release and working/tapping the spinal reflexes, should be applied first to the right foot and then to the left.

Inside edge of the foot – lumbar spine release ('banana')

Place yourself sideways on to the client's feet and put your palm over the top of the right foot so your fingers grip under the instep on the inside of the foot. Place your left palm firmly on top of the foot to steady it (usually with your finger pointing towards their toes). Firmly tuck the fingers of your other hand under the arch, and pull gently upwards as if to make a 'banana' shape. Hold for a few seconds and repeat three times.

Do not move or work the fingers that are hooked under the arch – they are simply being used as a lever to stretch the instep. Take care not to overbalance the client. The action of pulling the foot upwards a fraction, which I liken to pulling on a bowstring to fire an arrow, stimulates the spinal reflexes and can often ease low back pain quickly. Do not exert undue pressure on the tendon.

Reminder: key steps

- Approach the feet from the side.
- Support the top of the foot with one hand, grip the instep and pull gently upwards with the other hand.
- Do not move your fingers under the instep.
- Now work and tap the spinal reflexes described below then repeat the movement three times on the other foot.

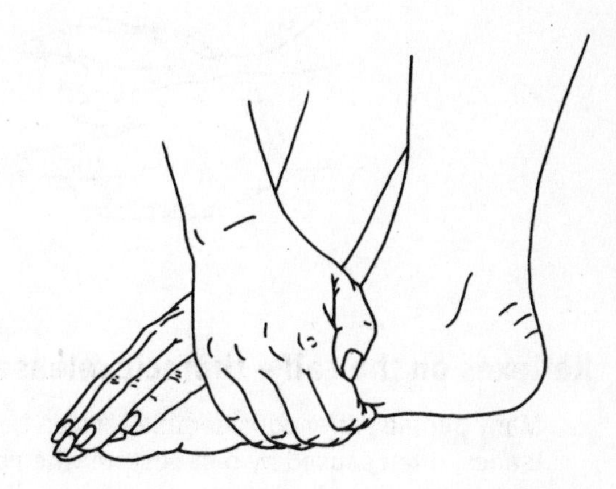

Inside edge of the foot – spinal reflexes

Work your index finger up and down the spinal reflexes using conventional reflexology techniques. Another equally efficient way is to place your hand so your palm covers the top of the foot and the index finger touches the cervical reflex points (on the side of the big toe). Then move all four fingers simultaneously down the spinal reflexes, pressing each reflex, until your little finger reaches the sacrum/coccyx reflex. Repeat three times. It is also helpful to 'tap' the individual spinal vertebra points with four fingers simultaneously from toe to heel (or heel to toe) three times, as it can stimulate the central nervous system. This is an extremely invigorating general tonic. Either move to the other side of the person or get them to turn and face the other way. Repeat these three movements on the left foot.

Reminder: key steps

- Work your index finger up and down the spinal reflexes.
- Caterpillar walk with your index finger and/or use your four fingers to work down the length of the spinal reflexes.
- Repeat three times.
- Tap up and down the spinal reflexes with four fingers three times.
- Ask your client to turn and face the other way, and repeat these moves and the 'banana' movement, on the left foot.

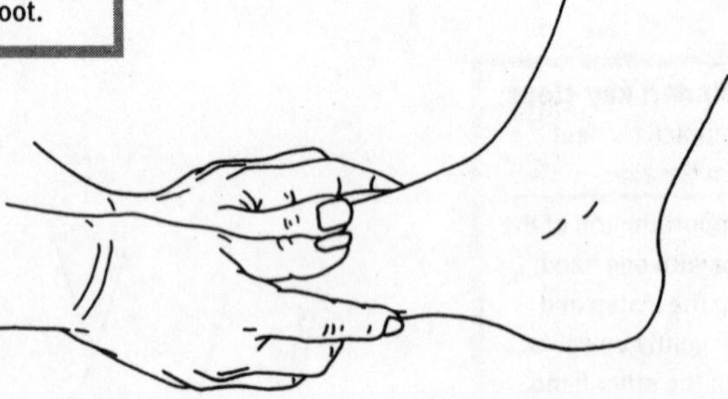

Reflexes on the calf – thoracic release

Many people suffer considerable tension between the shoulder blades, often caused by bad posture when driving or sitting. The back and ribcage can also feel very constricted if someone is suffering from respiratory problems or asthma. Unusually, I have found that there are a series of reflex points in a circle around the mid-calf. Often there can be an almost instant release of tension, and the person standing will feel a rush of warmth from their feet to their head as their back muscles begin to relax. They often report feeling quite sleepy and light-headed. Completely avoid touching varicose veins or a thrombosis.

Using two hands on the right leg pinch gently, and press once or twice, the reflexes on the entire circumference of the leg in the middle of the calf muscle. Repeat this procedure on the left leg.

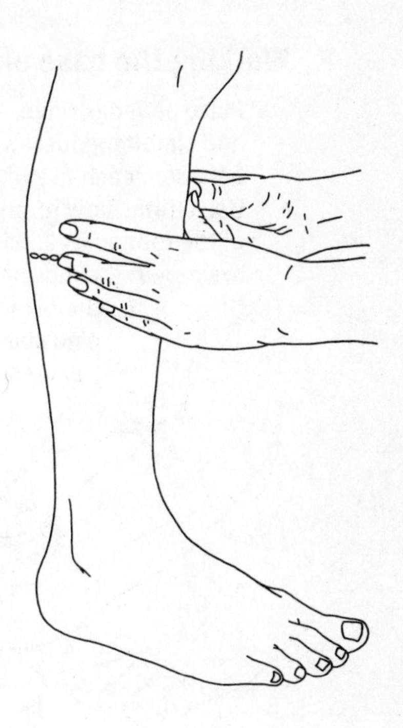

Reminder: key steps

- Locate a point on the mid-calf.
- Work using a fairly casual pinching and pressing movement with your fingers and thumbs, eventually treating the entire circumference of the leg.
- Work this mid-area once or twice so that all reflexes on this 'band' have been gently pressed and pinched. Then proceed to the other calf and repeat.

Working the toes – head area

The toes on both feet can be worked simultaneously. Kneeling in front of the client's feet, place your right hand on their left foot and your left hand on their right foot. Start at the big toes. Pinch, work and rotate your fingers on each toe individually, ensuring that the tips, sides and top are all contracted. The brain, sinuses, ears, eyes, neck and thyroid gland are all triggered when the toes are worked, as well as tiny subtle reflexes connected with the teeth, larynx and throat.

Reminder: key steps

- Kneel in front of the feet.
- Work both feet simultaneously starting from the big toes.
- Ensure that the sides and top of each toe are stimulated.
- Do not prise the toes apart if they are rigid.
- Pinch and work the feet gently to stimulate important head reflexes.

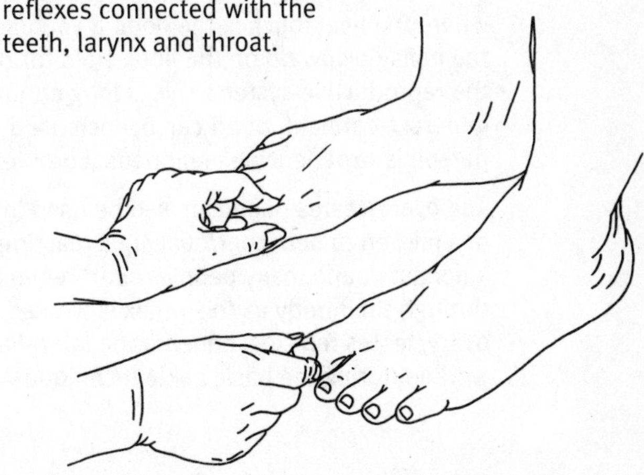

Working the base of the toes – lymphatic rotation

Place an index finger, or two fingers, at the bottom of both big toes and simultaneously work the lymphatic reflexes at the base of, and between, each toe where they join the metatarsal part of the foot. Use a firm, slow rotating movement, which circles the chest/lung area of the foot as well. When you reach the area at the base of the little toe repeat the movement from the opposite direction, returning to the big toes to finish. Not only is this movement pleasant and relaxing, but it gives the immune system a tremendous boost.

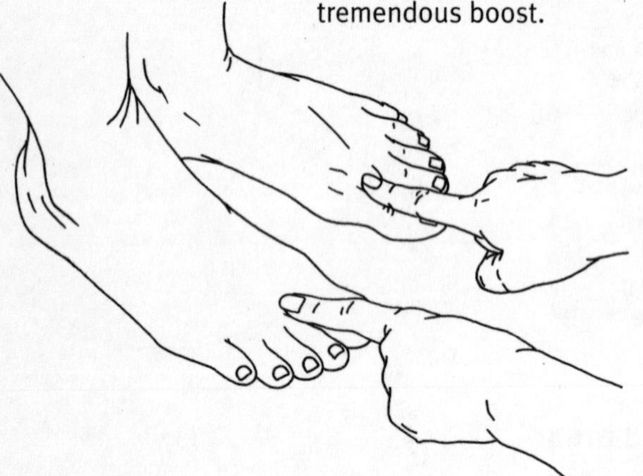

Reminder: key steps

- Work both feet simultaneously.
- Rotate the index fingers at the base of each toe and work the whole length of the foot, including the chest/lung area where the toes join the metatarsals (long bones on the main part of the feet).
- Repeat the movements in the opposite direction.

The base of the heel – ovary/testes helper reflex

Face the back of the heels and, using thumb, knuckle or index finger, firmly press the centre of each heel simultaneously at the point where the heel touches the floor. If you use your index fingers, place the nails downward on the floor. Hold for thirty seconds to balance the reproductive system. This is long enough if you are giving a general treatment, but it can be increased to forty-five seconds if the person is experiencing menopausal problems, for example.

The ovary/testes point can also be used in a totally different context on children to help control allergic reactions. This point is also an 'energiser', and many people report feeling warmth or tingling through their body as this reflex is worked. The conventional ovary/testes reflexes, beneath the lateral ankle bone, are routinely worked during the basic ankle techniques (see p. 94 and below).

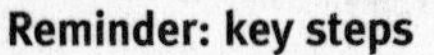

Reminder: key steps

- Firmly press the centre of heel at the base and hold for thirty seconds.

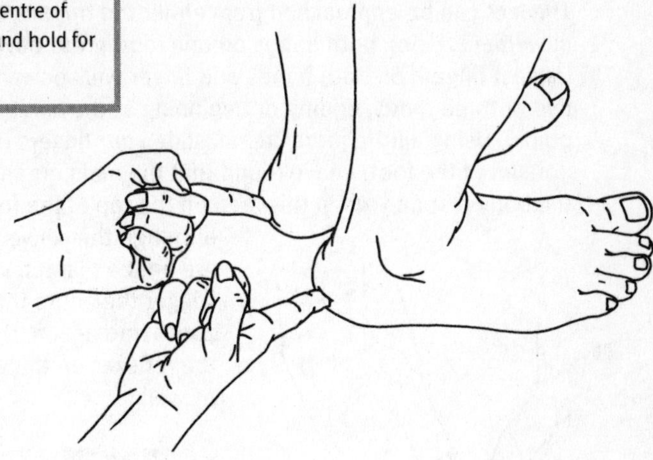

Return to the ankle reflexes

At least once during the VRT treatment return to the groin, pelvic, bladder reflexes etc. on the ankles. Press firmly into the groin reflexes and rotate, with your thumb or finger, around the ankle band. This movement appears to access new reflexes called Zonal Triggers (see Chapter 7), plus others which are connected with the heart and diaphragm. Working this area as described produces considerable relief and easing of tension.

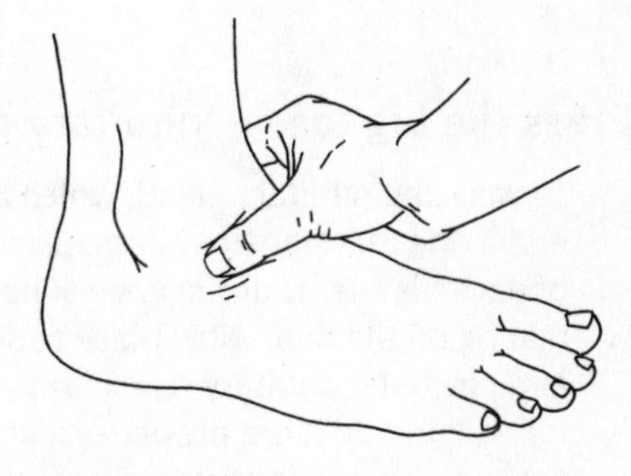

Finger walk the top of the foot (metatarsals)

The feet can be approached from either the front or behind for this movement. Using both hands on one foot, press down the three longest fingers on both hands and finger walk down the metatarsals two or three times, ending or beginning at the ankle groin/fallopian points. Using a little more cream, slide your fingers up and down the dorsum of the foot. I have found that the main organs and glands of the body respond when this area on the top of the foot is worked, although the conventional reflexes are on the plantar. VRT appears to trigger the entire three-dimensional zones into action, thus energising the reflexes on the sole of the foot as well.

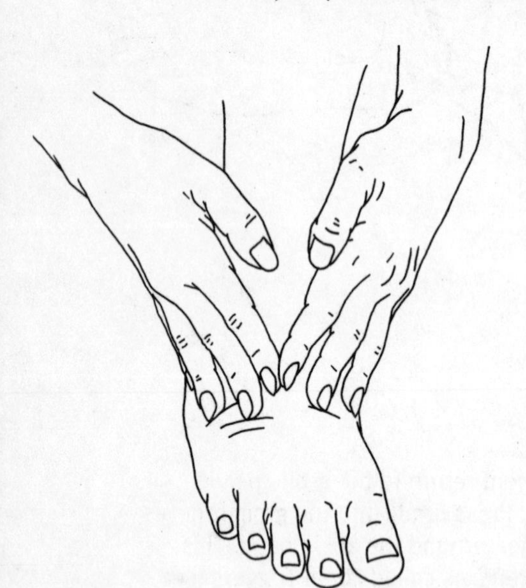

Reminder: key steps

- Use both hands either side of the ankle to work on one foot at a time.
- Move the fingers swiftly down the metatarsals from ankles to toes or vice versa.
- Make sure every part of the dorsum is stimulated two or three times, as this action is also treating every organ and gland in the body.

Press the big toes – 'pituitary pinch'

To work the pituitary gland, which is the master gland of the endocrine (hormonal) system, place an index finger under the centre of each big toe. Your fingers will be pressing upwards, with your nails resting on the floor. Now place your thumbs on top of each toenail and pinch the pituitary reflex firmly. Ask the client to lean very slightly forward to add more pressure, and hold firmly for thirty to forty seconds. This is an extremely powerful reflex point that helps to stabilise hormonal imbalances in both men and women. It can also have a relaxing effect, often producing an instant feeling of warmth throughout the body.

Reminder: key steps

- Place the index fingers, nails downwards, under each big toe.
- Find the centre of each big toenail with your thumb and press firmly.
- Ensure that the person is supporting themselves as they gently lean forward a fraction.
- Press both reflexes simultaneously for 30 seconds.

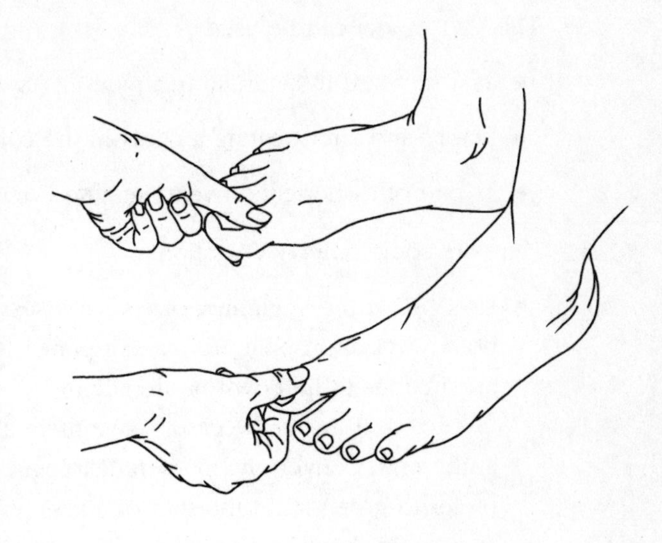

Variations

The treatment that you have learnt in this chapter is the model for all Vertical Reflex Therapy sessions. Once you have mastered the basics you will find it an extremely flexible treatment that can be adjusted to suit the time available and the client's requirements. Even if you forget the correct sequence always make sure you start with the ankle and spinal reflexes. Some of the techniques mentioned in passing have not yet been described and will be fully explained in the following chapters.

Let's now look beyond the model and examine variations and flexibility in methods of treatment once you become more confident.

- For chronic (long-standing) conditions work the reflexes twice weekly.
- Acute conditions can be worked daily if the schedule permits.
- Self-help VRT can be administered several times a day.
- Professionally it is usually impractical to treat clients more than twice a week. They can be taught self-help VRT techniques on the feet or hands to stimulate the immune system in between treatments.

The VRT model can be used

- as a standard five-minute treatment in its own right
- before and after treating a client in the conventional manner
- as part of a shortened twenty-minute Complete VRT Treatment.

Here are some other VRT options:

- Use VRT at the beginning or end of a session, but not both. It is not always appropriate to make a person stand on arrival if they are anxious to lie down or are talking and do not want to be distracted. If this is the case, I give them a few minutes of VRT at the end. Conversely, many reflexologists tell me that they prefer to give VRT at the start of a session because the client is so relaxed at the end that they do not want to disturb them.
- Give up to five minutes of VRT at the beginning of a treatment, and at the end just apply the extra Synergistic and Advanced techniques described in Chapters 7 and 8.
- Briefly work the ankles and the spine only at the beginning or end of treatment and immediately follow with two priority areas to treat synergistically, one three-point Zonal Trigger and optional Advanced Techniques.
- For real emergencies or on feet where I know the priority reflex points well I ask the person to stand and, after working the ankles and spine very briefly, I press two reflexes synergistically and one three-point Zonal Trigger as described in Chapter 7.

Vertical Reflex Therapy Basic Instructions

Do not treat with VRT for more than five minutes maximum in any one session, without the break of conventional reflexology in between. The maximum time would normally be five minutes at the beginning and two or three minutes at the end of a treatment. Often two or three minutes at the beginning and one minute at the end is all that is required to obtain results. The longest I have ever treated a client for is five minutes at the beginning and four minutes at the end of a session.

Basic treatment step by step – remember to keep alternating the feet!

1. Client is standing straight. Chair/table available to steady.
2. Always work ankles first! Start with either foot. Work hip/pelvic/ sciatic areas.
3. Slide/press/brush thumb across the top of ankle (fallopian tube reflexes) on each foot several times.

   Work 4a, b and c on right foot and then on left foot

4. **a** 'Banana' – move sideways to the feet. Press downwards on the foot with the palm of your hand, grip the instep and pull gently upwards three times.

   b Spinal reflexes: press vertebrae reflexes from toe to heel with thumb, index finger or four fingers – work reflexes three times.

   c Tap up and down medial side of foot three times each. Then work the other foot in same way.
5. Pinch round mid-calf circumference – thoracic reflexes. Two hands on one leg.
6. Kneel in front of feet: work toes on both feet simultaneously, starting from the big toes.
7. Press lymphatic reflexes at the base of all toes in a rotating movement. Work both feet simultaneously.
8. Return, at least once, to the ankle points to energise the body.
9. Press ovary/testes helper reflexes at the base of heel simultaneously for thirty seconds.
10. Metatarsals or main top part of the foot – work from behind the ankles to the toes with two hands – one foot at a time.

Synergistic Reflexology (Chapter 6)

11. Select two priority reflexes and work the hand and foot simultaneously.
12. Always work the same reflex area on both hands and feet to balance even if it is a right-or left-sided problem.
13. To conclude: 'pituitary pinch'. Pinch both big toes simultaneously. Client leans forward to exert more pressure.

Key points to remember

- Surroundings: have a chair or table to hold on to, and a quiet work room with no telephone to cause distraction.
- Equipment: towel to stand on, antiseptic wipes and non-oily cream (optional), plus a pair of hands with short, neat fingernails!
- Check there are no contra-indicated problems such as varicose veins on the calf, or a thrombosis. For general contra-indications see p.69.
- Make sure you are comfortable at all times as you work. Get the person on whom you are working, if they are able, to turn round so you can work the feet in different positions rather than you having to keep moving.
- Always start with ankle reflexes and keep alternating the feet.
- Remember to support the foot firmly with your other hand whenever possible.
- Return to the ankle reflexes at least once during a treatment.
- VRT can be a very pleasurable and gentle experience but it can also be momentarily quite painful. Tune into your client's needs and be ready to back off and work more gently. There can be gain without much pain.
- Don't forget the important concluding 'pituitary pinch' for about thirty seconds.
- Photocopy your Basic Instructions on page 103 and put it in a clear plastic folder or laminate it so that it remains clean and legible.
- Always warn a client that they may feel energised but equally they may feel tired or thick-headed after a treatment. This is a sign that the body is working hard to heal and detoxify itself.
- Advise everyone to drink more water generally, but especially after a treatment, to flush out the toxins and help prevent headaches.

Hand and Synergistic Reflexology (SR)

WHEN REFLEXOLOGY IS MENTIONED PEOPLE TEND TO THINK ONLY OF THE FEET. Often they do not realise that the hands can be as important and have as many reflexes. It is a great shame that most reflexologists spend little time learning about Hand Reflexology during their training. The same reflexes on the feet can be located on the hands, although there are anatomical differences in shape and size. The hands are not so physically sensitive as the feet, although they are much more accessible, but the reflexes *do* have the same energetic response as the feet.

What is Synergistic Reflexology?

Hand Reflexology has a vital role to play in accelerating the effects of VRT. It is a means of turning up the power in the body by simultaneously working two corresponding reflexes – one on the hand and one on the foot. I call this technique Synergistic Reflexology because the impact of working two identical reflexes, for example the hip/ankle and hip/wrist points, at the same time produces a more effective result than if I had worked the two reflexes separately. The word 'synergy' means the increased effect achieved by having two factors working in co-operation.

The aim of working two reflexes together synergistically is to help channel extra healing energy towards a particular organ, gland or limb. As the hand contains all the same reflexes as the foot, it is just a question of familiarising yourself with the hand charts and observing the anatomical differences between the hands and feet. In Synergistic Reflexology you simply find the same points on the hand as you have found on the feet and work the two together for a maximum of thirty seconds.

Having learnt the Basic VRT method in Chapter 5 you are halfway to synergistic work already. Once you have mastered the Hand

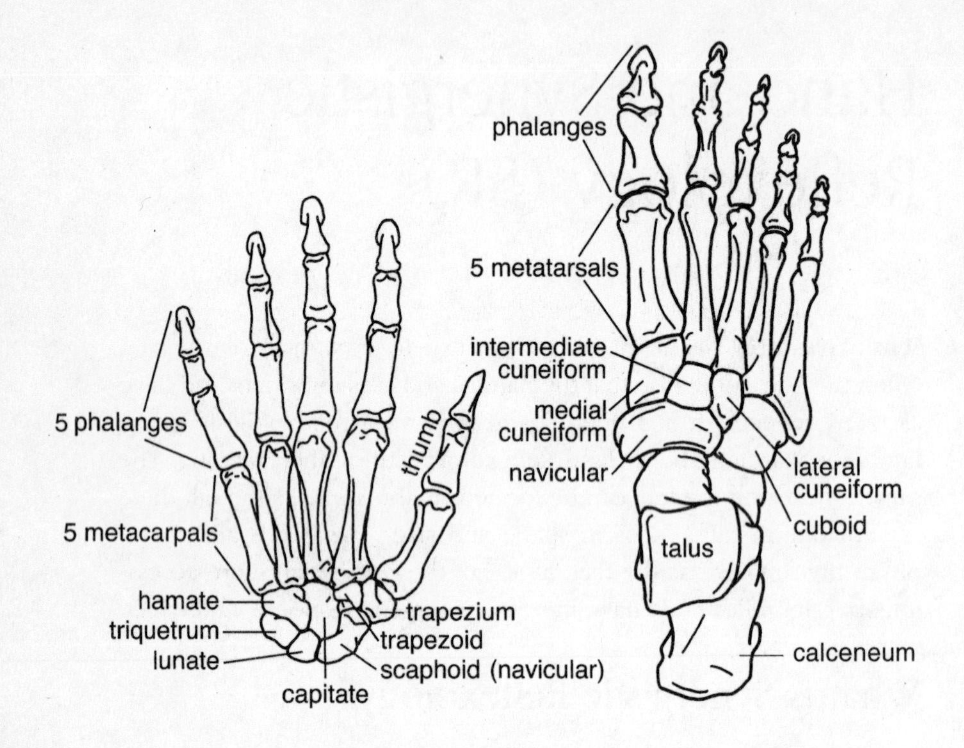

Reflexology instructions in this chapter you will have enough information to enable you to practise effective Synergistic Reflexology. If your reflexology training was purely about the feet, or you wish to pursue hand techniques further, practical courses for working the hands are available through reflexology schools. One excellent pioneer is reflexologist Kristine Walker, author of a definitive book called *Hand Reflexology*. Kristine's work and research have shown that the hands are just as receptive to reflexology as the feet. When she used hand reflexology on post-operative hip replacement patients their general recovery was much quicker than that of patients who did not receive reflexology.

This chapter will explain exactly how to work the standing feet and hands together. You do not need to be a contortionist or have to stretch to practise SR, as the client's arms will be hanging down beside their body with their hands only a few centimetres above the knee. Fortunately VRT is a very short treatment, taking only one to five minutes, so you can sit or kneel comfortably on the floor as you simultaneously press a foot and hand reflex. A small cushion is useful to sit or kneel on.

Synergistic Reflexology takes the separate benefits of hand and foot reflexology three stages further by:

- working the same reflexes on the hand and foot simultaneously when the client is reclining or standing
- working the hands alone – pressing the palm downwards on a table so that it is weight-bearing and then work the hand
- simultaneously working the weight-bearing hands (palm downwards) and the standing feet.

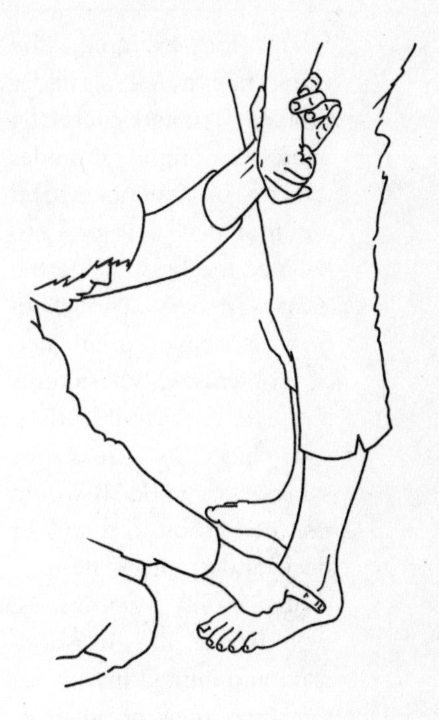

Working two reflexes synergistically

The scope of working a maximum of three reflexes synergistically per session

Working the hand and foot reflexes together for a minute or two is not arduous, as it takes only a short time to simultaneously work a maximum of three points on each foot in any one treatment – or two Synergistic points and one Zonal Trigger as described below. They must be the same three points on each foot to keep the body in balance. If, for example, you work the liver, on the right foot, you should still work the same part of the foot/zone on the other foot to balance the body, even though there is no corresponding liver reflex on the left foot. This is a very important rule when working on the standing feet. Why? Because the body is being stimulated to send extra energy to parts that have a priority requirement, and if this energy is sent in too many directions at once it not only dissipates the effect but tires the body. The aim therefore, is, to decide which parts of the body most need help.

If, for example, the client had a left shoulder problem, I would still briefly work the right shoulder reflexes on the right hand and foot as well, in order to balance the body using the Zonal Triggers. The client may also have complained of problems with her uterus and eye, so I would prioritise these as areas for synergistic work. I would *not* then go on to work her neck and stomach reflexes synergistically, because I would have already prioritised and limited myself to the three areas of greatest need.

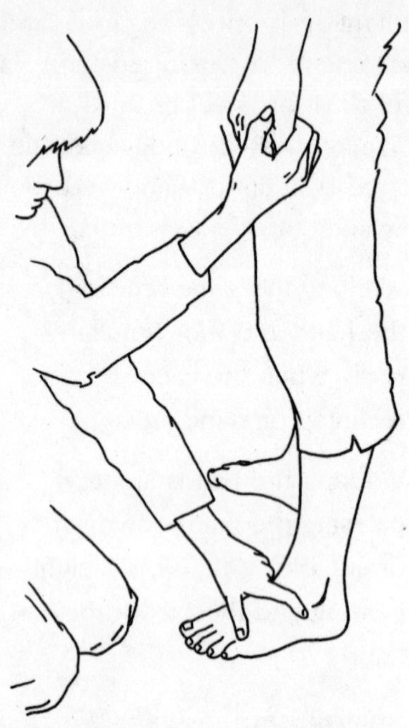

Working three reflexes simultaneously

The use of Diaphragm Rocking, described on p. 116 and 119, will ensure that you have got it right, because the gentle rocking movement pumps energy to where the body needs it most. Usually any reaction in the body will correspond to one of the priority reflexes.

Hand reflexology

The basics of VRT and Hand Reflexology can be examined with reference to the hand charts opposite. For VRT and SR you do not have to learn much about the hands to be successful! Your only requirement is to find a maximum of three reflexes on the hands to work synergistically – you do not treat the entire hand. The hands would only be given a full treatment if Weight-bearing Hand VRT, described on p. 113, was applied. Then you would work the entire top of the hand as the client pressed their palm downwards to rest on a table.

Position your hands carefully

When working on a client's hands, using VRT or SR, it is essential to position your own hands so as to exert the correct pressure, without placing any strain on your hands.

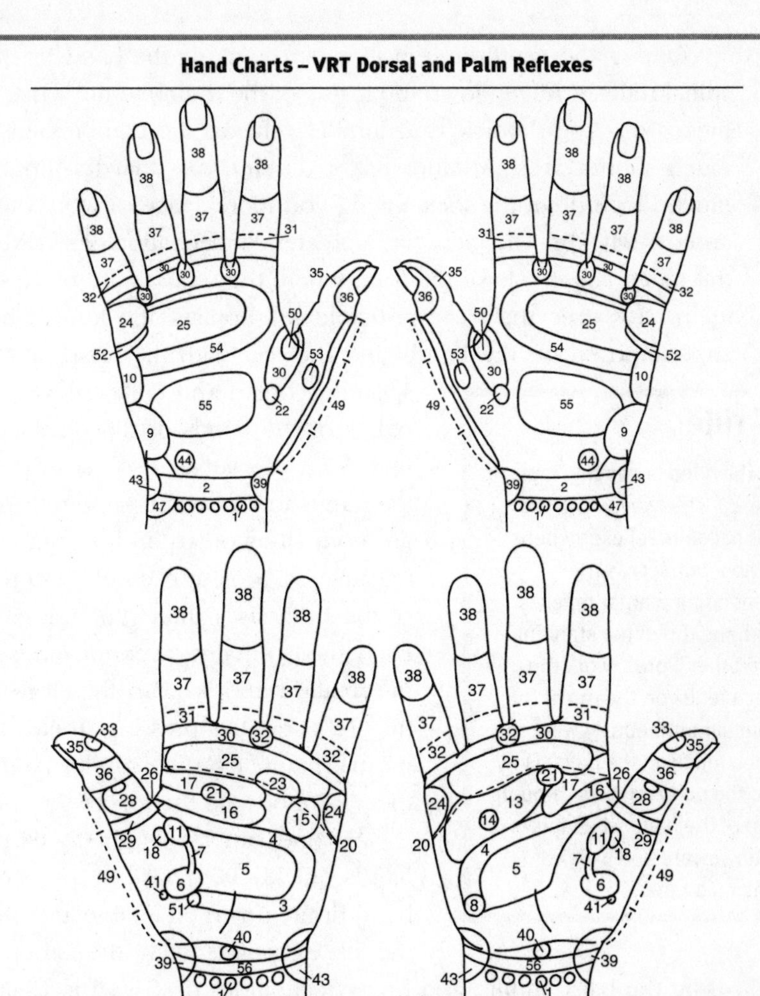

Note: All palm reflexes can be accessed via the dorsum of the hand when weight-bearing.

1. Zonal Triggers
2. Fallopian tubes/ seminal vesicles/vas deferens/ groin/lymphatic/helper diaphragm/heart
3. Sigmoid
4. Colon
5. Small intestine
6. Bladder
7. Ureter tube
8. Appendix/ileocecal valve
9. Knee
10. Elbow
11. Kidney
13. Liver
14. Gall bladder
15. Spleen
16. Pancreas
17. Stomach
18. Adrenals
20. Diaphragm
21. Solar Plexus
22. Thymus
23. Heart
24. Shoulder
25. Chest/lung/breast
26. Trachea/oesophagus/ bronchial tubes
28. Thyroid/parathyroid
29. Neck
30. Lymphatics
31. Eyes
32. Ears/Eustachian tube
33. Pituitary/pineal/ hypothalamus
35. Brain/skull
36. Face/teeth/ jaws/ tongue/ throat
37. Helper sinuses/teeth
38. Sinuses/brain/skull
39. Uterus/prostate
40. Helper ovary/testes
41. Penis/vagina
43. Ovary/testes
44. Hip sacro/ileac joint
47. Hip/pelvic area
49. Spine
50. Larynx/vocal cords
51. Anus/rectum
52. Armpit
53. Breastbone
54. Ribs
55. Mid/lower back
56. Sciatic nerve

One of the main differences when working the hands is that the spinal reflexes travel down the inside of the thumb to the wrist, which means that the thoracic and lumbar reflexes are compressed into a much shorter area. Another major difference is that the fingers are much longer than the toes, giving you more space to work the sinus and ear reflexes. The palm has a greater concentration of reflexes than the much larger sole of the foot, where the reflexes are more spaced apart. However, the basic principle still applies: the human body is superimposed on the hands and the feet with the torso and corresponding organ and limb reflexes on the palms of the hands or the plantar of the feet. VRT, of course, also uses the top of the hands to access the same reflexes that are normally worked on the palm. This is because we look at each of the ten zones of the body as a three-dimensional slice. Each slice contains layers of reflexes and information and we can therefore access the reflexes by pressing them in the normal manner on the sole or palm or in the VRT mode on the top of the foot.

VRT rule

When the hand is hanging loose in standard VRT, always work the traditional palm reflexes where applicable but access the corresponding plantar reflexes through the top of the standing foot. In other words, work the stomach reflex on the top of the foot but simultaneously work the stomach reflex on the palm. Only access the palm reflexes through the top of the hand when it is palm downward and weight-bearing on a table.

Anyone can be taught to treat their hands quickly with VRT by pressing one hand firmly down on a table and working the reflex points with the other hand, using the basic thumb and finger techniques described in Chapter 4. The stomach, kidney and all other organs can all be worked through the back of the hand. Carers can also be taught to work another person's hands, and it provides a shared treatment for partners or for the infirm who cannot kneel on the floor to treat someone's feet. Chapter 9 describes self-help techniques on the hands and feet (see diagram p. 148).

Four ways of accessing a correct hand reflex

1. Consult the Palm Reflexes Hand Chart (on p. 109) and use your fingers and thumb to locate the palm hand reflexes on a friend's or your own hands, and practise the basic finger pressure reflexology techniques that were taught in Chapter 4.

2. Now place your hand palm downwards and weight-bearing on a table and locate the Dorsal Hand Reflexes, on the top of your hand, with your other forefinger and thumb. (See Dorsal Hand Chart on p. 109.) Palm reflexes can be accessed via the dorsum.
3. If at any time you do not have a Hand Reflex Chart available but are familiar with the reflexes of the foot, then study the hand carefully and locate on it an area that roughly corresponds to a foot reflex you wish to treat synergistically. Work this area, and concentrate on any reflexes that seem tender. For instance, the eye reflex at the base of the third right toe could be tender, so you would locate the eye reflex on the hand by working the base of the third right finger. You will often find that there is a tender spot on the hand that links to a similar point on the feet.
4. The simplest method of Synergistic Reflexology: you can give an holistic five-minute VRT treatment in which your attention is simply focused on working the entire foot and hand with no reference to any particular reflexes. However, you may find the same three tender reflex points on each foot and then work the corresponding areas on the hand, which may or may not feel tender. Once these two points are located the reflexes should be worked for a maximum of thirty seconds simultaneously.

One interesting aspect of VRT and SR is that the hand reflexes can suddenly become much more tender when the corresponding foot reflex is worked at the same time. SR stimulates the hand reflexes to become even more sensitive after they have been held for about thirty seconds. Many reflexologists initially think that the hand reflexes are less sensitive than the feet. They are not – there is just a slightly slower response.

Guidelines for hand reflexes

The wrist corresponds to the ankle, the fingers to the toes, the palm to the sole, and the heel of the palm to the heel of the foot. It is only the spine and neck reflexes that need closer examination, as they are not so similar. The spinal reflexes on the hand run from the outer side of the thumb to the wrist, whereas the foot spinal reflexes run from the edge of the big toe to the heel.

Working the hands conventionally

If you cannot work the client's feet for any reason, you will still be able to treat the hands conventionally and in a weight-bearing position. A conventional Hand Reflexology treatment should take about thirty to thirty-five minutes. First relax the client's hands by gently massaging them with both your hands, using a very small amount of non-oily cream. Place their elbows on a cushion, on a table for support, with their palms facing upwards.

Palm:

Use the standard thumb technique to inch across the palm so that every reflex is stimulated. Keep working across the palm from different angles to cover every part. Make sure your other hand is firmly holding the client's hand so that it is well supported.

Fingers and thumbs:

Use your forefinger to work down the tops of the client's fingers from the nail of each finger and thumb in a rotating movement to the base. Work down both sides of each finger and the thumb as well. This enables the finger reflexes on both sides to be worked at once.

Top of the hand:

Place the client's palm in your own palm for support and work the top of their hand with your thumb. Work in all directions to cover all the reflex points, and try inching across the top of the hand (dorsum) pressing the reflexes with your four fingers.

Webbing of the hand:

Pinch the webbing between the thumb and forefinger and between the fingers. Your thumb will be pinching the palm as you pull your thumb and forefinger across this loose fleshy area of the hand. This accesses the reflexes for the neck and throat as well as those for the eyes and ears.

Wrist band on the hand:

Slide and then work your thumb across the top of the wrist several times. You can also make little 'caterpillar bites' with your forefinger as this will stimulate the groin, fallopian tube and new helper heart and diaphragm reflexes, as well as the Zonal Triggers.

Weight-bearing hand reflexology using VRT techniques

When the client's hands are placed palm down, arms straight, on a table the same weight-bearing principles of foot VRT apply to the hands:

- Work both hands for a maximum of five minutes in all.
- Work the top of the hands to access all the palm reflexes (see the VRT Dorsal and Palm Hand Charts on p. 109). Stimulate the reflexes using the basic finger and thumb techniques explained in Chapter 4.

Follow this sequence and remember, if you are not working on yourself, to alternate the hands from time to time to keep the body in balance. Throughout the treatment the hand(s) being worked should remain on the table.

Wrists (1):

Starting with the client's left or right hand, work the side of the wrists first to treat the hip/pelvic/sciatic reflexes. The ovary/testes and uterus/prostate reflexes are also worked.

Wrists (2):

Slide/press/work your thumb across the top of the wrist on each hand to work all the reflexes including the deeper Zonal Trigger points.

Inside or medial edge of the hand (1):

The 'banana' movement eases the lower lumbar spine. Move sideways to the client's hands. Press the top of their hand downwards with your palm, and with your other hand place your index and third finger under the client's palm – nails downwards, below the bottom thumb joint, and give a gentle pull upwards. Do this three times per hand.

Inside edge of the hand (2):

Remain sideways-on to the client's hands and continue working the spinal reflexes. Press the vertebrae reflexes from thumb to wrist with your thumb or fingers three times, then tap up and down the spinal reflexes three times using your fingers.

Mid-arm:

Using your two hands to work one arm, pinch round the circumference of the arm midway between the wrist and the elbow to stimulate the thoracic reflexes.

Thumbs and fingers:

Facing the client's hands, work the thumbs and fingers on both hands simultaneously. Start at the thumb and rotate your index fingertip on the top of each finger. Then pinch along the sides of the fingers, ending at the little fingers.

Base of fingers:

Starting at the thumb, work the lymphatic reflexes by rotating on both hands at the same time. Work the base of all the fingers in a rotating movement using two fingertips, circling the fingers over the chest/lung reflexes.

Wrist points:

Return, at least once during the treatment, to energise the body by means of the Zonal Trigger reflexes.

Ovary/testes reflexes:

Simultaneously press these helper ovary/testes points, which are located at the mid-point on the heel of each wrist, with your index finger for thirty seconds. These are situated in the middle of each palm where the wrist and palm join. You have to stretch slightly behind the arm to reach these points.

N.B. The conventional ovary/testes reflexes are situated on the outside edge, or lateral part, of the hands at wrist level. These can also be worked now to consolidate the treatment.

Work the top of the hand:

Work across the metacarpals upwards from the base of the fingers to the wrists, using your two hands to work each of the client's hands one by one. Make three passes over each hand, moving your fingers in tiny bites of pressure on the reflexes as you progress.

Select up to three priority/relevant reflexes:

Select reflexes appropriate to the person's condition, and work hand and foot reflexes synergistically for thirty seconds per reflex.

Conclude with the pituitary pinch:

Pinch both thumbs simultaneously, making sure that your thumb covers the client's nail and your index finger is placed directly underneath the tip of the client's thumb to cover the pituitary reflex. Hold for thirty seconds.

Synergistic reflexology and weight-bearing hands

The weight-bearing feet and hands can be worked synergistically for a few seconds if you are treating an intractable problem. But it is not easy to work the hands and feet at the same time when the hand is weight-bearing because it is situated further away from the practitioner and you have to stretch at an odd angle to find the reflex points. I only use this method if the person has not previously responded to VRT, especially if they are suffering from orthopaedic or mobility problems, as these conditions react particularly well to VRT in general and to double weight-bearing in particular.

Synergistic Reflexology is usually applied to the weight-bearing feet and the loosely held hands because it is easy to apply and the response is excellent. The bony top of the hand is more difficult to work when weight-bearing but can still be effective. A person who is wheel-chair bound or unable to stand may still have enough strength in their arms to place their hand on a low stool beside their chair. They can then firmly press their palm downwards and in this instance their hand, not their foot, receives VRT.

Zonal Triggers (ZT) and weight-bearing hands

The Zonal Triggers are a row of tiny, powerful new reflexes that are situated round the wrists and ankle bracelets. By brushing and working the thumbs across these points a healing response is triggered through all the zones to every part of the body. In Chapter 7 the role of the Zonal Triggers on the feet is discussed in detail. If you work the hands in a weight-bearing position, and exert pressure on the hand reflexes and the Zonal Triggers, the client can feel the sensitivity on these points increase as the cumulative effect of working three reflexes together takes place.

At this point, however, all you need to know is that there are important new Zonal Trigger (ZT) reflexes and that they are stimulated by brushing and working the thumbs across the wrist on the back of the hands. This brushing technique also works the standard groin and fallopian tube/*vas deferens* points, plus the helper heart and diaphragm reflexes on the wrists.

The hands and Diaphragm Rocking (DR)

Diaphragm Rocking is a profound technique which pumps energy to the part of the body which is most in need of stimulation at any particular moment. It usually consists of a rhythmic rocking of the feet but can also be used on the hands, and is described in detail in Chapter 7. A unique feature of DR is that it allows the body to prioritise where to send an energetic impulse regardless of which reflexes have been previously worked. Often a feeling of warmth or tingling accompanies the surge of energy through the body. DR is extremely effective on the feet and helpful on the hands, although it is often difficult to fully support the arm and smoothly rock the hand unless the arm is resting on a cushion. Hand DR can be used halfway through a conventional thirty-minute hand treatment or at the end of a brief five-minute VRT session if the client is unable to recline and have their feet rocked.

Diaphragm hand rocking

1. Sit the client opposite you across a small table, with their right or left arm resting on a cushion or towel in front and their palm downwards.
2. Allow their elbow and lower arm to remain on the cushion, and lift the hand so the palm is facing you and the fingers are pointing upwards.
3. Place both thumbs horizontally to the heel of the hand on the diaphragm line and centred on the solar plexus reflex.
4. Place the four fingers of both hands on top of the client's hands so that they make a V-shape, with your fingers pointing towards their wrist.
5. Rock the hand backwards and forwards to test the range of its mobility without straining. Press the metacarpals firmly and slide your fingers outwards a fraction to 'fan' and stretch the metacarpals as the client's hand is pulled down towards you.
6. As soon as the hand is pulled forward, take the pressure off the metacarpals, press the solar plexus reflex with your two horizontal thumbs and push the hand back towards the client.
7. Once a rhythm is obtained, rock gently at least fifteen times per hand. This should be visualised as a pumping action, with energy being pumped round the body to the area of greatest need. It is helpful to count 'one and two' as you push forward and 'three and four' as you pull towards you. You can continue these actions for two to three minutes. Hand DR is useful, but foot DR is exceptional.

Key points to remember

- Synergistic Reflexology, like all VRT techniques, can also be used frequently in conventional treatments when the person is in a reclining position. It still produces subtle benefits but, if the feet are not weight-bearing, it is not as powerful.
- Because SR is much less powerful when the feet are not weight-bearing you can treat as many parts of the body as is necessary – not just three priority reflexes.
- SR can be worked on two priority reflexes in any one session. Select the second and third areas of the body in most need of help. The top-priority reflex will be worked using the SR techniques and a third point on the ankle – the Zonal Trigger.
- Always work the same reflexes on both feet, even if the problem is only on one side of the body. This balances the body and helps the general equilibrium.
- Work reflexes simultaneously on both feet/hands for thirty seconds each.
- Do not underestimate Hand Reflexology – it is a very powerful and profound tool for practitioners to use.
- Study the hand charts carefully, they have a different emphasis to the feet, as the proportions in the structure of the hands place the reflexes in a slightly altered relationship to each other.
- Teach your friends and clients to work their hands between treatments. Hands are far more accessible and discreet to work in public, and easier for the elderly and carers to work.
- If you have a particularly intransigent problem and SR does not help, try working on the weight-bearing hand and foot at the same time. This is not as easy to administer as when the client's arm is hanging down beside them, but can be very successful.
- Be conscious of the extra sensitivity in the hands when the hand and foot reflexes are worked simultaneously. The hand reflex becomes much more tender within seconds of the SR technique being introduced to the corresponding foot reflex.

The Complete VRT treatment

including Diaphragm Rocking, Zonal Triggers and Lymphatic Stimulation technique

TWO BENEFICIAL ASPECTS OF VERTICAL REFLEX THERAPY ARE ITS FLEXIBILITY AND quick application. We have already covered Basic VRT in Chapter 5. This chapter is about Complete VRT, a comprehensive twenty-minute session in which conventional reflexology is sandwiched between two brief VRT treatments.

Most reflexologists are content to include VRT at the beginning and end of normal treatments that usually last between thirty and sixty minutes, and this is the way I usually use it myself. However, Complete VRT places the emphasis on VRT within the context of a much shorter standard reflexology treatment where the client is in a reclining position for only ten or twelve minutes. During that time only the sole or plantar of the foot is quickly worked, and halfway though that treatment Diaphragm Rocking (DR) and Lymphatic Stimulation (LS) are introduced.

At this stage many therapists may be asking how such a short treatment can be complete or effective. It is effective because the weight-bearing VRT at the beginning and end accelerates the energy to the vulnerable parts of the body and, given the impressive results achieved after a five-minute Basic VRT, it is not surprising that the whole treatment is enhanced. The soles can be very precisely worked in ten minutes because the rest of the foot has already been treated with VRT. The Advanced Techniques in Chapter 8, and those which will be described in this chapter, are also quick and easy to incorporate into this short treatment as a way of fine-tuning the body.

Enhancing VRT

The effectiveness of VRT is enhanced by the Diaphragm Rocking (DR) technique, which was introduced in Chapter 6 in relation to hands (see p. 116) and is applied to the feet when the body is in a reclining position. The Zonal Triggers (ZT), also introduced in the previous chapter (see p. 115) work in conjunction with the hand reflexes. They add a third, very powerful dimension to VRT because they enable three reflexes to be worked at once: two on the feet and one on the hand. In other words, ZT takes Synergistic Reflexology one step further.

Basic Lymphatic Stimulation (LS) is the final new technique to be learnt in this chapter. It is a simplified version of a very powerful series of movements devised by my colleague Hedwige Dirkx, who teaches VRT in Belgium and Holland. The lymphatic system, as explained in Chapter 2, is a drainage system for the circulation, and the lymph nodes play an important part in removing toxins from the body and increasing immunity. The technique taught in this chapter stimulates the abdominal lymphatic system on the soles of the feet following Diaphragm Rocking. It takes only a few minutes on the reclining feet and is relaxing, soothing and beneficial to all conditions.

Diaphragm Rocking, Zonal Triggers and Lymphatic Stimulation are simple techniques to learn but have a profound effect on the body's own healing mechanism. Once you have learnt them they can be incorporated into the Basic VRT treatment you learnt in Chapter 5.

'How can a professional reflexologist regard Complete VRT as comprehensive when it takes only twenty minutes?'

Looked at in terms of results, Complete VRT is truly comprehensive. This is because the entire body is worked thoroughly and effectively due to the concentration of power in the reflexes. Indeed, many therapists obtain better results from twenty minutes of Complete VRT than from an hour of standard reflexology. Complete VRT is not designed to totally replace hourly reflexology treatments where the client can truly relax. It simply offers a very efficient option.

Diaphragm Rocking (DR)

I devised this technique originally to combat insomnia, as it was very good at resetting the body clock. In fact, DR was so effective in this respect that I began to receive phone calls from people who were not remotely interested in reflexology or its many benefits and just wanted me to rock their feet. I discovered that DR could indeed work in its

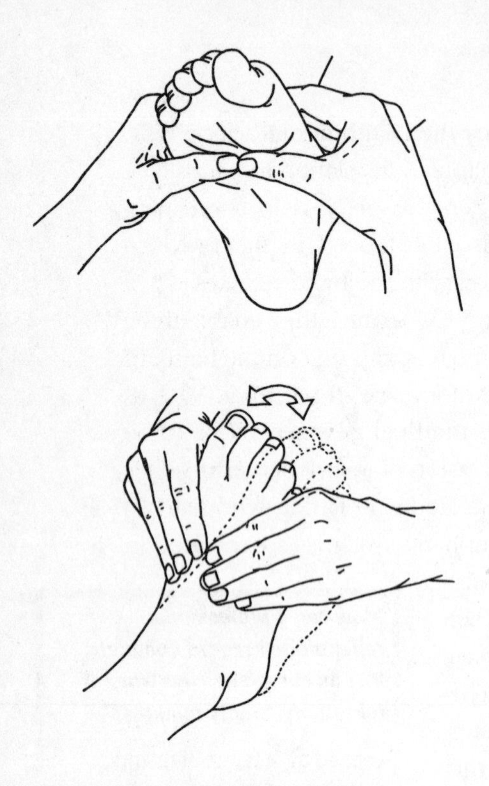

Diaphragm Rocking technique

own right if administered to someone lying in bed ready for sleep, but this is only appropriate for family and friends.

After I had been using VRT extensively for a year I began to think about the wider potential of Diaphragm Rocking. I reasoned that, if it could balance the sleep patterns in the body, it could probably help the equilibrium and healing of the body in general. This point appeared to be proved quite rapidly. Halfway through a treatment I would begin my rocking technique and assumed that relief would be felt in the areas I was working such as the solar plexus reflex. To my surprise, clients and volunteers said they were feeling warmth in various parts of their body. Often it would be in the throat or chest area if they

Case study

Darren was a forty-six-year-old plumber who had hurt his back lifting a heavy water tank. He came for VRT after the osteopathic treatments, on which he usually relied, had not helped this time. He had pain in his right forearm and left buttock, and limited rotation to the left in his neck. The general discomfort meant he was also sleeping badly. He was given Complete VRT, which included working on the Zonal Trigger for his neck and Diaphragm Rocking to help balance his body alignment. Afterwards he immediately had more movement in his neck and reported feeling quite light-headed. Over the next few weeks he had two more treatments and the pain and restricted movement slowly cleared, until he suddenly noticed that it had disappeared completely. He returned for another Complete VRT treatment a few months later when he said he felt the problem was starting again and he wanted to nip it in the bud.

Case study

I had been treating a middle-aged woman for a dry ticklish cough that would not abate. She had suffered from mild bronchitis a month before and, although she felt fully recovered, she kept coughing at night due to a 'tickle in her throat'. The neck and throat reflexes were tender and I worked them well with various VRT techniques. Her chest/lung area on the foot felt clear, so I concentrated on the upper respiratory tract reflexes. When I gave her Diaphragm Rocking she almost immediately relaxed her diaphragm and her breathing became deeper as I rocked each foot in turn. As I was completing the movement on the second foot she suddenly sat up and choked and asked for a tissue. For a moment I thought she was going to be sick, but instead she coughed up a thick lump of mucus that had obviously been irritating her lungs for some time. Despite my experience I had not found the correct reflex, but DR had allowed the body itself to prioritise the part most in need and then extra energy was channelled in that direction. The following day the woman rang to say her cough had virtually gone and she had slept through the night.

were stressed, but occasionally it would be in the weak spot in their body.

Although I was concentrating on the rocking and trying to help the client, I often became aware of warmth in my own chest and would feel calm and relaxed. I have concluded that this gentle rocking, over a period of one to four minutes, sets up an exchange of neutral energy between the therapist and the person treated that is powerful and relaxing to both. I use the term 'neutral' because a therapist must not take on the negativity or angst of their patient any more than they dump their own stuff on unsuspecting persons who pay for a treatment!

Since that time the rocking movement has been extremely helpful in cases of trauma, deep stress, addiction and chronic illness that will not respond to conventional, or at times complementary, treatments. It can be used in every reflexology treatment, whether VRT is introduced or not. In my opinion the effect of DR is as profound as the effect of VRT. Both accelerate the healing properties that lie within the body. Zonal Triggers, Synergistic Reflexology and other techniques enhance VRT, but Diaphragm Rocking appears to over-ride, if necessary, the key reflexes that a reflexologist has chosen to work.

Diaphragm Rocking Method

Diaphragm Rocking is applied about midway through the VRT/reflexology treatment when the person being treated is very relaxed and in a reclining position.

1. Always ensure that the feet are facing you as straight as possible and do not force them outwards as you work. If the feet naturally splay outwards they should be allowed to do so, but keep them as straight as is comfortable while you administer the rocking movement. Do not use extra cream on the feet for DR.
2. Position both thumbs horizontal to the heel under the diaphragm reflex, meeting at the solar plexus point.
3. Place your four fingers of both hands on top of the foot, so that the fingertips touch and the index fingers form a 'V' which points towards the ankles.
4. Gently rock the foot back and forward to test the range of its mobility from the ankle. This is a pleasant treatment, so the foot should not be overstretched or pushed back on itself to make the ankle feel uncomfortable. Press only on the solar plexus reflex as the foot goes forward towards the client.
5. The pressure on the solar plexus reflexes and the top of the foot should be firm and equal. Most therapists can push firmly on the sole of the foot but are inclined to put too little pressure on the metatarsal bones as the foot comes towards them.
6. As the foot comes towards you, the pressure on your thumbs is released and your fingers press the top of the foot firmly. It is essential at this stage that your fingers do not slide away from the middle of the foot or squeeze it. Slightly stretch the metatarsal bones apart on the top of the feet as the foot rocks back towards you.
7. Once a rhythm is obtained, continue to rock at least fifteen times per foot. With some conditions, or for deep relaxation, you may rock each foot for up to two minutes – four in total.
8. Make sure you sit upright in your chair as you work and allow your elbows to bend outwards as you push the feet. It is deeply relaxing and calming for both practitioner and client.

Case study

For several months I had been treating Wendy for menopausal hot flushes, lower backache and asthma. Sometimes I would work other reflexes synergistically – if she had a cold I might work the sinus points instead of the spinal reflexes, or if she had diarrhoea I would work the colon. On arrival she had a few minutes of VRT and Synergistic Reflexology and then relaxed on the couch while I worked her feet. About halfway through the treatment I always gave her Diaphragm Rocking. One day I had given her SR on her back, uterus and chest, yet when it came to the Diaphragm Rocking she touched her lower abdomen and said her bladder area had 'gone all warm'. I asked if she had a urine infection or similar problem, and she said she had not. On her next visit she rather sheepishly remarked that she had been experiencing stress incontinence for a few weeks, but had been too embarrassed to tell me that every time she coughed or laughed she involuntarily passed a small amount of urine. Since that feeling of warmth in the bladder/urethra area the problem had much improved. It was interesting that, despite my concentration on three priority areas for SR, the body had over-ridden my intention and sent energy and healing to the area of real priority at that particular time. Working the lower back would have also helped the spinal nerves which send and receive messages to and from the bladder.

Diaphragm Rocking is so relaxing that many therapists ask why I do not recommend using it at the beginning of a treatment. There are two good reasons. First, it is important that the person does not relax too quickly as the therapist needs some feedback as he or she begins to work the reflexes. Some of them can be tender, and the therapist needs to know what immediate effect the treatment is having. Second, many reflexologists do not like their clients to fall asleep as they feel it detracts from the treatment, though personally I feel that it is their time and they must use it as they wish; if they are very tired, the body is allowing them some rest in the day. The best solution is to work the feet system by system and then introduce Lymphatic Stimulation and Diaphragm Rocking halfway through the treatment. The client often relaxes so quickly and deeply that he or she cannot help but fall asleep or at least doze.

Zonal Triggers (ZT)

Vertical Reflex Therapy has opened up a new way of accessing the body's own healing mechanisms through the deeper set of reflexes on the ankle and wrist bands that I have called Zonal Triggers. These are a series of tiny reflexes that form a circle round the ankles and wrists and can only be accessed when worked in conjunction with other specific reflexes on the hands and feet. When I discovered these different reflexes I found that the tiny pin-prick sensation on the ankle was nearly always situated in the same zone as the corresponding reflex.

I often use the analogy that Zonal Triggers work in rather the same way as an electricity junction box. It contains a row of fuses (reflexes) that enable power to travel round the house (body) via the wiring (the zones). If a light goes out somewhere in the house (a part of the body is malfunctioning) we have to go to the junction box (ankle band reflexes) to locate the fuse (reflex) and replace it (work it to bring back the power). ZT and Diaphragm Rocking are the most powerful tools in fine-tuning and regenerating the body when using VRT.

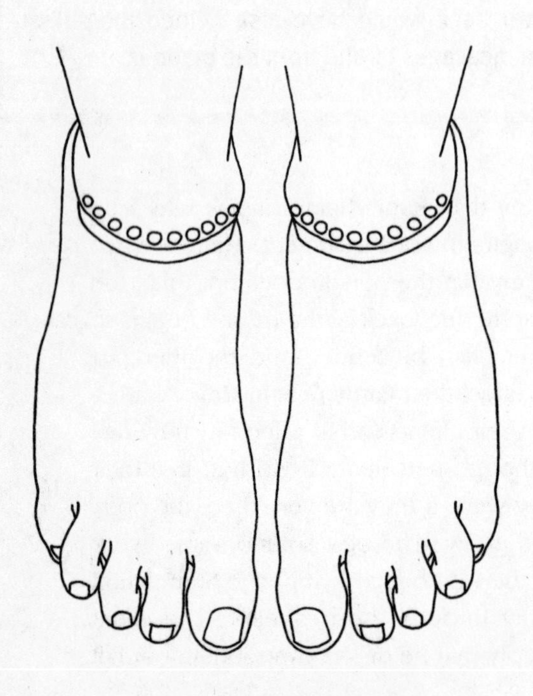

Position of Zonal Triggers on ankle

The VRT ankle reflexes are an extremely important 'window' into the body, and many orthopaedic conditions respond quickly when the Zonal Triggers on the ankles are worked. These same reflexes round the ankle (conventional fallopian tube reflexes) respond at a deeper level when the person is standing, causing the heart and diaphragm to respond.

Having discovered these special reflexes I began to try to map them out. Fortunately I soon realised that this method was flawed, and I would not need to

Case study

Lucy, twenty-seven, came to me for reflexology because she had suffered for months from splitting headaches. She also had a very stressful job and her neck and shoulder reflexes were very tender. When taking her case history I asked her if her bowel function was normal and she replied that it was, although as I worked the soles of her feet the colon reflexes felt rather rigid. At the end of the session I asked her to stand for VRT. I worked the colon and lumbar spine reflexes synergistically, then placed my index finger on a neck reflex and carefully felt round the ankle in zone one for the appropriate ZT. I could not find one, so I worked further round the ankle until I found a reflex that felt like a sharp pin-prick when I touched it. It was in zone three, so I worked the neck and the ZT in zone three for thirty seconds per foot. The same tender reflexes in zone three along the sole and the top of the foot related to the colon in Lucy's case. I again asked her if she had bowel problems such as constipation, as many headaches are caused by digestive problems especially in the colon. She said no, and told me that she regularly passed a motion every four days as that was the norm for her! In subsequent treatments I used a ZT on the neck or colon reflex, depending on which was more tender, but the ZT was always in zone three and not zone one for the neck. Gradually the constipation and headaches improved with VRT and conventional reflexology, aided by the fact that I encouraged Lucy to drink more water and make a few dietary changes. This is an interesting example of how the Zonal Trigger indicated the root cause of a problem and guided the therapist to look further than the problem as it was presented.

draw up complicated charts and try to get reflexologists to remember every reflex. The reason it was unsatisfactory was that sometimes the pin-prick sensation was not in the corresponding zone to the reflex I was working but further round the ankle. I had told colleagues to work a point in the same zone as the corresponding reflex if they could not find a pinprick point anywhere, and this advice still applies. But what if there was a tender spot elsewhere – should that be worked instead? The answer is yes, because it can indicate that another function or part of the body is affecting the malfunctioning organ, bone, muscle or gland. Occasionally there may be more than one pin-prick point. If so I always work the one in, or nearest to, the corresponding zone to the reflex.

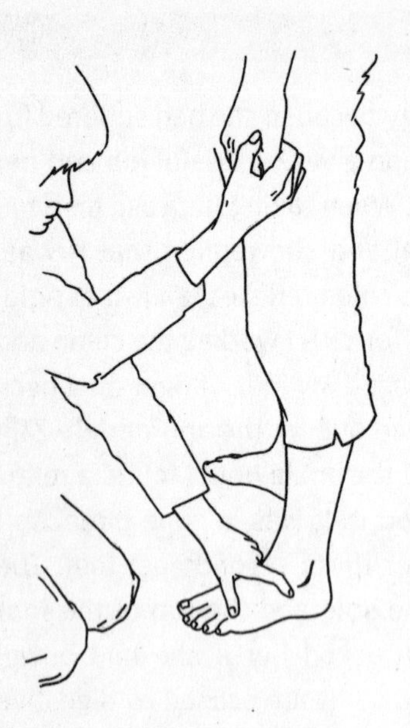

Shoulder problem – Working the hand and foot reflex synergistically plus the appropriate Zonal Trigger

The Zonal Triggers place greater emphasis on the power of Hand Reflexology and Zone Therapy, the precursor to reflexology which still forms a major part of its theory. This theory states that the body is divided into ten longitudinal zones – five on each foot. There are also three transverse lines across the feet, which mark the areas that mirror the shoulder girdle, waistline and pelvic floor in the body. The flows of energy throughout the body are directed through these ten zones. VRT appears to decongest the zones very quickly, allowing energy to flow through unimpeded.

The ZT reflexes should be visualised as one of two deeper layers of reflexes on the ankle or wrist band that are positioned below the conventional reflexes as follows:

Top layer of reflexes:

Conventional lymph and groin/fallopian tube/*vas deferens*/seminal vesicle.

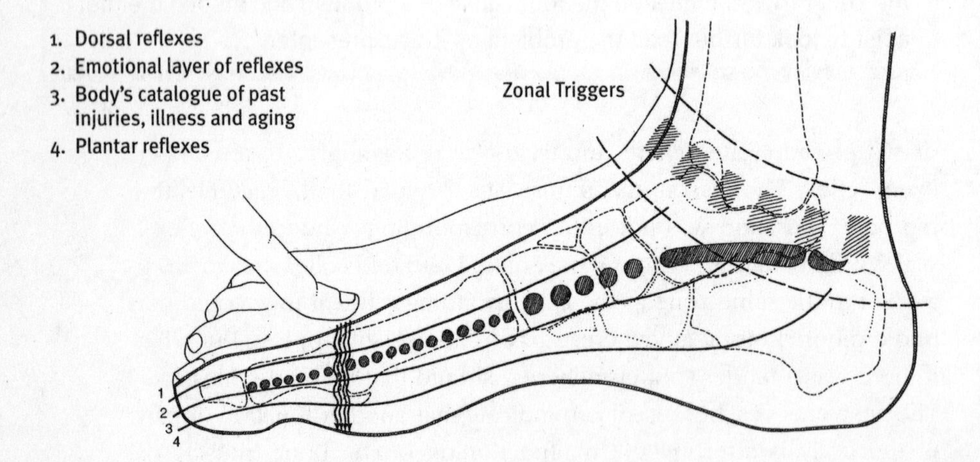

Cross-section of foot illustrating the three-dimensional aspect of four layers of reflexes

Middle layer of reflexes:
VRT helper diaphragm (left and right foot/hand) and helper heart (left foot/hand).

Deepest layer of reflexes:
The Zonal Trigger reflexes that are activated when worked simultaneously with another reflex that relates to a specific part of the body. They appear to allow energy to flow through the zones unimpeded, resulting occasionally in an instantaneous response from an organ, gland, muscle or part of the skeletal system. Working these three points at once has such a powerful effect that the stimulation can often bring about very quick relief from long-term conditions.

Prioritising a reflex using Zonal Triggers

Working the ZT is an extension of Synergistic Reflexology, in which the same hand/foot reflexes are worked simultaneously. Once the appropriate hand and foot reflexes have been located a third reflex is located around the ankle; then two points are worked on the foot while a third is worked on the hand. These triggers work by increasing the power, or stimulation, from the reflexes to the condition most in need of treatment. Let's use the uterus/prostate reflex as an example. You can use either hand, whichever is the more comfortable, to locate the reflexes.

1. Kneel or sit beside the client in a comfortable position. Locate the uterus/prostate reflex below the inner ankle on the right standing foot – although it does not matter which foot you start with. As with Synergistic Reflexology, next locate the corresponding hand reflex which, in this example, is on the inner edge of the wrist.
2. Work the right hand and foot reflexes synergistically for a few seconds.
3. Temporarily let go of the hand and continue to hold the reflex on the foot. With your other hand work your index finger or thumb round the ankle band in tiny 'bites', starting at the back of the foot above the heel. At some point, usually in the same zone as the reflex you are pressing, the client will feel a tiny tender pin-prick. This is the Zonal Trigger.
4. If you fail to find a ZT in the corresponding zone keep working round the foot until you locate a pin-prick spot and hold it. If there is no

tender point, return to the correct zone in line with the priority index and hold that point instead with your index finger. If you find more than one pin-prick reflex of equal intensity work the ZT that is most in line, preferably in the same zone, as the key reflex on the foot.

5. Then press the ZT reflex with your index finger. Use it as a pivot for your hand, so that your thumb touches the uterus/prostate reflex on the right foot, and hold the two.
6. Now reach up and relocate the uterus/prostate reflex on the wrist. Hold the three points together for thirty seconds.
7. Repeat on the left foot and hands in the same manner. Always work the same reflexes on both feet to balance the zonal energy (the energy that runs through a particular zone). Even if it is a one-sided problem, such as the left shoulder, always work the corresponding reflex area on the other side of the body to balance. Never work two different ZTs on the right and left foot because it is very unbalancing and negative for the body – there is a conflict of interests as the body tries to focus on two priority points.

Zonal Triggers in the reclining position

If the client is in a reclining position it is perfectly acceptable to work several ZTs during one treatment, as long as both feet are worked each time, because the energy is subtle and not so powerful as when standing. Even if it is a one-side problem, work the same area/zone on the other foot to balance the body's energy.

Use the Zonal Triggers during every treatment, whether conventional or VRT, to enhance your results. Do not work a reflex for longer than thirty seconds. The reflexes can be rotated or held still with slight pressure.

Lymphatic stimulation (LS)

This technique can be used before or after Diaphragm Rocking and can be applied for up to two minutes per foot. The combination of stimulating the abdominal lymph system in conjunction with working the weakest reflexes is a powerful new tool for reflexologists. Ideally, LS and DR should be introduced roughly halfway through a treatment, as the body will have been treated with VRT and conventional reflexology and is more responsive at this stage. With the permission of its originator, Hedwige Dirkx, I have abstracted the following technique.

Method

The aim is to use the thumbs on the soles of the feet in a sweeping movement from the outside or lateral part of the foot. Each movement stimulates the reflexes that affect the abdominal organs, and the sweeping movements are designed to increase the flow of lymphatic fluid to help cleanse the body.

1. As the client lies in a reclining position, place one thumb on the sole of each foot, in the area of the liver reflex on the right foot and the spleen area on the left.
2. Press your thumbs firmly into the soles of the feet. In a sweeping movement make an arch with your thumbs across all the abdominal reflexes, ending in the area of the lumbar spine.
3. Repeat these sweeping movements several times so that the thumbs start a little nearer each time to the outside of the foot and finish further down the lumbar spine, nearer the heel of the foot. The treatment should take about one to two minutes.

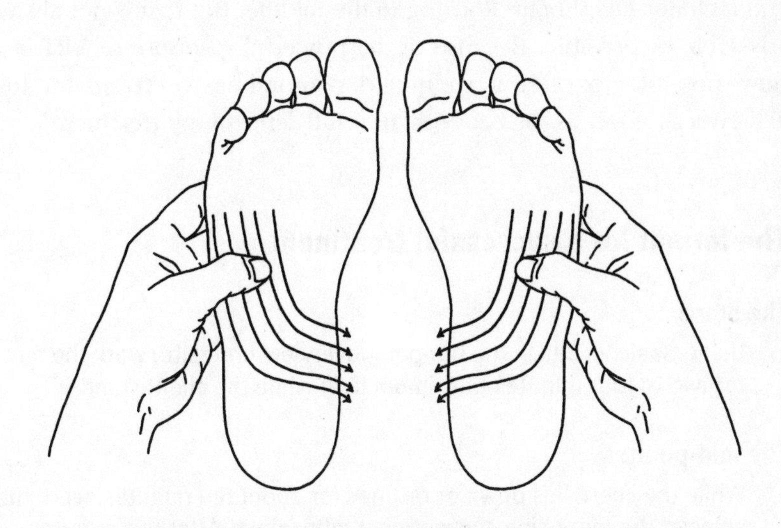

Lymphatic stimulation – always work in a medial direction

This is a rudimentary but effective treatment when used in conjunction with VRT and reflexology. Reflexology is one of the best methods of assisting lymphatic drainage in the body and there are excellent specialist courses run by reflexologists for those who want to develop the techniques further (see p. 184).

Complete VRT – brief twenty-minute treatment guide

We are now going to look at a model treatment for Complete VRT which you can use as a blueprint for future treatments. This short but extremely comprehensive treatment should last about twenty minutes. I will also indicate where the strict order of treatment is essential for good results and good health, and where you can freely adapt it to your own needs and those of your client.

In this and previous chapters you have learnt both Basic VRT and the fine-tuning techniques of Synergistic Reflexology, Diaphragm Rocking, Lymphatic Stimulation and the Zonal Triggers. All of these can be worked on the reclining feet as well as the standing feet, the latter being more powerful.

Nothing can be better than a full reflexology session of thirty to sixty minutes that encompasses some VRT at the beginning and end and includes Diaphragm Rocking in the middle. But that is not always advisable or possible. Because of the powerful response of VRT, it is now possible to offer a shortened comprehensive treatment that achieves as good as, or better than, a full reflexology treatment.

The format for a successful treatment

The start:

Using Basic VRT as in the ten-point overview opposite, work the feet for two to four minutes (maximum five) while the client stands.

The mid-point:

While the client lies down or reclines for about ten minutes, work the soles of the feet using conventional reflexology. After five minutes introduce Lymphatic Stimulation for a minute or two, followed by approximately one to two minutes of Diaphragm Rocking. Then resume working on the second foot or continue working the systems of the feet one by one.

The conclusion:

The client stands again and you quickly rework the pelvic reflexes round the ankles and the spinal reflexes on each foot for a few seconds to stimulate the zonal energy.

Then work two reflexes on each foot synergistically. Work the corresponding reflexes on both feet even if it is a one-sided problem.

Then locate the priority reflex relating to the weakest part of the body synergistically on the hand and foot. Find the pin-prick Zonal Trigger on the ankle and hold the hand reflex simultaneously while your thumb and finger hold the two reflexes on the feet for thirty seconds each foot.

Ten-point recap of Basic VRT

Remember to keep alternating the feet. Start with either foot. The areas *printed in italics* must always be worked first.

1. Client stands straight. Have a chair/table available on which to place a hand to steady (full sequence Chapter 5).
2. *Always start on ankles first! Work hip/pelvic/sciatic area around ankles.*
3. *Slide/press/brush thumb across top of ankle band on each foot.*
4. *Three movements on one foot, then change to other foot.*
   - (a) Spinal 'banana' movement – move sideways to the feet. Press top of foot, grip instep and pull gently upwards – three times per foot.
   - (b) Spinal reflexes. Press vertebrae reflexes from toe to heel with thumb or forefinger three times.
   - (c) Tap up and down spinal reflexes three times.
5. Pinch/press mid-calf circumference – thoracic reflexes. Two hands on one leg.
6. Kneel in front of feet. Work toes on both feet simultaneously. Pinch sides.
7. Work/rotate lymphatic reflexes on both feet at base of all toes once or twice.
8. Return at least once to ankle points to energise the body.
9. Press helper ovary/testes point at base of heels simultaneously for thirty seconds.
10. Metatarsals – work from behind the ankles with two hands towards the toes – one foot at a time.

Re-cap of 'fine-tuning' techniques and their place in Complete VRT

Diaphragm Rocking and Lymphatic Stimulation:

- Two essential soothing and rocking techniques, in the reclining position, for mid-point in every reflexology treatment.

  To end Complete VRT swiftly work both ankles for a few seconds and then apply the following techniques:

Synergistic Reflexology (SR):

- Select up to two priority/relevant reflexes appropriate to the person's condition. Work hand and corresponding foot reflexes simultaneously for thirty seconds per reflex.

Case study

Malcolm is an engineer in his late forties who had fallen down a flight of stairs while carrying heavy equipment and had hurt his back, neck and shoulders. A few weeks later he attempted to lift a heavy barrel of fluid into his van and his lower back seized up under the strain. He had been in agony for a week and was on strong painkillers when he limped into my clinic unable to rotate his neck or bend his back. I worked on him with VRT for about four minutes at the start of the treatment and then gave him some conventional reflexology. He found lying down for any length of time very uncomfortable. At the end of the treatment I once again got him to stand as best he could and repeated the Basic VRT technique for another three to four minutes, followed by SR on the neck and shoulders and ZT on the lumbar spine. As I pressed the ZT points he gave a gasp of pain and bent double, and we both thought his back muscle had gone completely into spasm. In fact it had released, and he was immediately able to stand up straight with very little pain – just a residual soreness. This was an exceptional result, and I was able to work the two VRT treatments of about four minutes each in the same treatment because it was an acute injury and the working of the reflexes in a standing position was not continuous. It was broken up by a session of conventional reflexology.

I have since occasionally used full Basic VRT twice in a reflexology treatment when treating acute injuries and have had excellent results, though not as spectacular as in Malcolm's case. His back improved immediately and there was no return of the acute pain.

Zonal Triggers (ZT):

- Locate main priority reflex on foot and same one on the hand. Work across ankle band to locate ZT which is usually, but not always, in same zone.
- Work/hold all three reflexes simultaneously for up to thirty seconds per foot. (NB The same reflex or corresponding area must be worked on both feet and only one 3-point ZT should be used per treatment.)

At this point some Advanced Techniques from Chapter 8 could be introduced.

Pituitary pinch:

- To conclude, pinch both big toes simultaneously from pad to nail. Client leans slightly forward to exert more pressure.
- Hold for thirty seconds.

Variations on the Complete VRT treatment

When using VRT in a Complete Treatment the same options apply as in a full reflexology session. All these reasons below are valid and all methods are successful – the choice is up to the reflexologist.

Variation 1:

Use Basic VRT at the beginning of a session only, and include the SR and ZT work at the same time for five minutes. Always use DR and SR at the mid-point. Apply no VRT at the end of the session.

Reason for this mode of treatment:

The client is too relaxed to want to stand again, has to hurry off immediately the treatment is concluded, or the therapist wants to stimulate the body first so it responds better to conventional reflexology.

Variation 2:

Use Basic VRT at the end of a session only, and include SR and ZT for five minutes. Always use DR and SR at the mid-point.

Apply no VRT at the beginning of the session.

Reason for this mode of treatment:

The client needs to be made comfortable at once and does not want to stand for VRT on arrival, or the therapist wants to discover the priority reflexes before working with SR and ZT.

Variation 3:

Basic VRT is applied for a maximum of two to three minutes at the beginning and end of Complete VRT plus SR and DR mid-point. SR ZT and/or Advanced Techniques are then applied once only at the end of the treatment for about two to three minutes.

Reason for this mode of treatment:

This one is usually used on clients with acute problems or who have suffered accidents and the body is in trauma (see Malcolm's case study). Do not use it for chronic cases in your early treatments, as here the body needs a more subtle and shorter VRT treatment to allow time for gradual regeneration.

Variation 4:

Use Basic VRT for two to three minutes at the beginning and end of Complete VRT plus SR and DR mid-point. Work the weight-bearing hands and feet for the SR and ZT techniques. Follow with Advanced techniques if required.

Reason for this mode of treatment:

Intransigent problems that have not responded to VRT and need extra help.

Key points to remember

1. Do not underestimate the powerful response to the shortened Complete VRT Treatment.
2. When practising Complete VRT spend the ten minutes on conventional reflexology working the soles of the feet only.
3. Use the shortened treatment more often on family and friends – there are now fewer excuses that you haven't got time!
4. Use Diaphragm Rocking in every reflexology treatment, however long or short, and whether VRT is included or not.
5. Practise Diaphragm Rocking so that it flows smoothly and you too can relax and experience a neutral exchange of energy.
6. Increase the length of time spent on Diaphragm Rocking to a total of three or four minutes when dealing with deep trauma, emotional or physical.
7. Use the Zonal Triggers frequently in conventional treatments. Several different ailments can be treated when the client is in a reclining position.
8. Do not overwork the reflexes when using the Zonal Trigger – a maximum of thirty seconds per reflex is all that is required.
9. Use Lymphatic Stimulation technique as a general boost to the immune system in every treatment.
10. Explore new areas for using the shortened Complete VRT treatments such as schools, sports teams, hospitals, offices and voluntary work if you wish to adapt or expand your practice.

Advanced VRT techniques

THIS CHAPTER DESCRIBES OPTIONAL ADVANCED TECHNIQUES AND SKILLS TO USE during VRT treatments of any duration. All or any of them can be added to Basic VRT or Complete VRT, or can be used as part of a full VRT/conventional reflexology treatment. They can also be used on the weight-bearing hands. Some of these methods can also be freely used on the feet when the client is in a reclining position. They enhance VRT but are not an essential part of a treatment and tend to be used only by professional reflexologists, especially when the client has particularly complex health problems that are not responding to traditional reflexology or Basic VRT.

Only the ankle and spinal reflexes need be worked on the standing feet, to stimulate the Zonal Triggers immediately before applying advanced techniques. These methods can also be applied to the weight-bearing hands. This short cut can help limit the treatment time and is also helpful in keeping VRT treatments down to a maximum of five minutes at any one session. Remember that you can occasionally give four or five minutes of VRT at the beginning of a treatment followed by up to four minutes at the end, although it is rarely necessary to work so long using VRT. The body would be over-stimulated if VRT was used continuously for nine or ten minutes. The various techniques are:

- Extending the combination of reflex points to enhance VRT treatments.
- Stimulation of Neural Pathway reflexes and Zonal Triggers.
- Metatarsal Pressure on the cervical and spinal reflexes.
- Plantar Stepping – a subtle technique used for chronic conditions especially digestive.
- Knuckle Dusting – stimulation of the central nervous system and general toning techniques.
- Palming – a stimulating technique that is more gentle than Knuckle Dusting.

Extending the combination of reflex points to enhance VRT treatments

As you become more proficient in using VRT and the accompanying techniques, you will be able to decide which combination of methods and reflex points is most relevant for certain conditions. Sometimes a practitioner will begin to get results using VRT, DR and SR and then the client reaches a plateau and appears not to improve any further. It is then that the variations on VRT techniques can be utilised to help bring about a positive response. There are numerous permutations, some of which are listed below. It is assumed that Basic VRT will be used first, for one to four minutes, at the beginning or end of a session or both.

Examples of combination of Advanced VRT techniques

Synergistic Reflexology:

Simultaneously work the hand in a weight-bearing position as well as the foot. This is very helpful for orthopaedic and mobility problems that have not yet responded.

Zonal Triggers:

Work the neural pathway reflex on the spine while the foot is in the Metatarsal Pressure position. The extra weight/pressure on the ball of the foot seems to enhance the reaction of the reflexes. Link with the dorsal and ZT reflex and work the three points together for thirty seconds on each foot. This is useful when helping chronic conditions.

Knuckle Dusting and Palming techniques:

Use on the standing feet and then immediately repeat the actions on the top of the weight-bearing hands, palm face downwards on a table. This is particularly helpful for asthma and depression.

Plantar Stepping and Metatarsal Pressure:

Metatarsal Pressure places all the weight on the ball of the foot and increases the reflex response for neck, spine and shoulders. With Plantar Stepping, the client places one foot at a time at a 45 degree angle and the therapist pinches up and down the outside edge of the foot so the reflexes are simultaneously worked on the top and sole of the foot. At the same time the client can work the outside edge of their palm in the same way provided they have a chair near to steady

themselves if necessary. This can work well on digestive ailments, especially as the helper dorsal digestive reflexes are worked on the top of each foot overlapping zones 4/5.

Stimulation of the Neural Pathways (NP) and Zonal Triggers (ZT)

The body functions smoothly and healthily when the Central Nervous System (CNS) is working well. It is said that about 50 per cent of all health problems are related to spinal disorders or misalignment, and these problems do not manifest themselves just in painful back conditions. If the spine is compromised in some way, the functions of the central nervous system are also impaired. The spinal column protects the spinal cord, from which an array of nerves extend to specific parts of the body as shown on the simplified chart opposite. The function of the nervous system is to relay information between the brain and all parts of the body (see Chapter 2). If a spinal vertebra is slightly under pressure or has been damaged in an accident then organs and other parts of the body can be affected, because the information from the nerves is inadequate.

The aim of this technique is to fine-tune the working of the thirty-one pairs of cervical and spinal reflexes by simultaneously working the appropriate spinal vertebrae, each of which also contains a spinal nerve reflex, and the corresponding organ reflex on the hand or foot. Readers who are unfamiliar with the central nervous system and corresponding vertebrae should refer to the chart depicting the position of the neural pathways opposite. This technique can be used on a client who is in the reclining position.

- For best results use the knuckle or the outer edge of your thumb. Work down the spinal reflexes on the medial or inside of the foot until you come to the area where you would expect to find a certain reflex, e.g. small intestine, at the waistline (below the raised first tuberosity of the navicular bone). Consult the chart and work as precisely as you can to the vertebra reflex that corresponds to the organ.
- For example, the spinal reflex (T12) and the tender intestinal reflex should be worked simultaneously. The spinal vertebrae

Reflexologists' Spinal Chart

(see also illustration on p. 81)

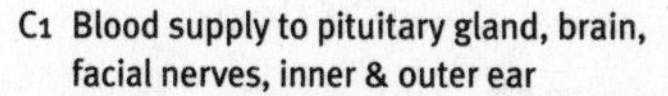

C1 Blood supply to pituitary gland, brain, facial nerves, inner & outer ear
C2 Eyes, sinuses, optical & auditory nerves, tongue
C3 Outer ear, cheeks, teeth, trifacial nerve
C4 Eustacian tube, centre face
C5 Vocal cords, neck glands
C6 Shoulders, neck muscles, tonsils
C7 Thyroid, elbows
T1 Fore-arms, wrists, hands & fingers, oesophagus
T2 Cardiac system
T3 Respiratory system, breasts & chest
T4 Gall bladder
T5 Liver, solar plexus
T6 Stomach
T7 Pancreas, duodenum
T8 Spleen, diaphragm
T9 Adrenals
T10 Kidneys
T11 Ureters, kidneys
T12 Small intestines, lymph
L1 Colon
L2 Abdomen, upper leg, appendix
L3 Reproductive system, bladder, knee
L4 Prostate gland, sciatic nerve, muscles of the lower back
L5 Lower legs, ankles feet and toes

SACRUM Hip bones, buttocks, bladder

COCCYX Rectum, anus

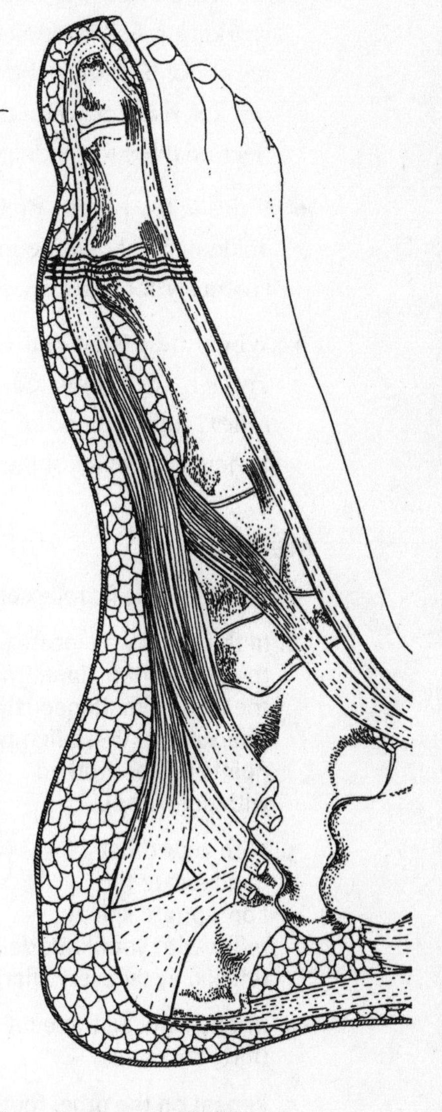

The spinal and neural pathway reflexes in relation to the foot

The Nervous System is extremely complex. This chart offers simplified guidelines for reflexologists and indicates links between the spinal vertebrae and some nerve inervations to various parts of the body. It does not purport to be a precise medical chart. Parts of the body are supplied by different sets of nerves such as the sympathetic and parasympathetic nervous systems and these nerves can stem from various parts of the spinal cord. The reflexologist can still work effectively when using VRT to stimulate the neural pathway reflexes by using the techniques described in this chapter. Results can be obtained by locating the distinct *pinprick* sensation on reflexes when a connection is made between the appropriate Zonal Trigger, nerve and body reflexes.

are marked on the foot charts and the exact reflex is found by working a few centimetres up and down the foot charts in the region of T12 until the most tender reflex is located. The pin-prick sensation when the organ and spinal nerve reflexes connect enables the therapist to work extremely accurately.

- If this is the priority problem for the client, the Zonal Trigger on the ankle band should be located and the three reflexes worked simultaneously for thirty seconds a foot while the client is standing.
- When the neural pathways, including the appropriate Zonal Trigger, are stimulated, the third reflex worked is a spinal foot reflex, rather than the actual hand reflex used in standard Synergistic Reflexology or ZT stimulation.

Method

1. Find the specific reflex on the top of the foot and work it briefly.
2. In the usual way locate and work the appropriate Zonal Trigger on the ankle simultaneously with the reflex point (these first two points will be worked with one hand).
3. With your other hand locate the appropriate spinal reflex with your knuckle, or side of the thumb, and work it firmly. The reflex may feel very sharp or painful.

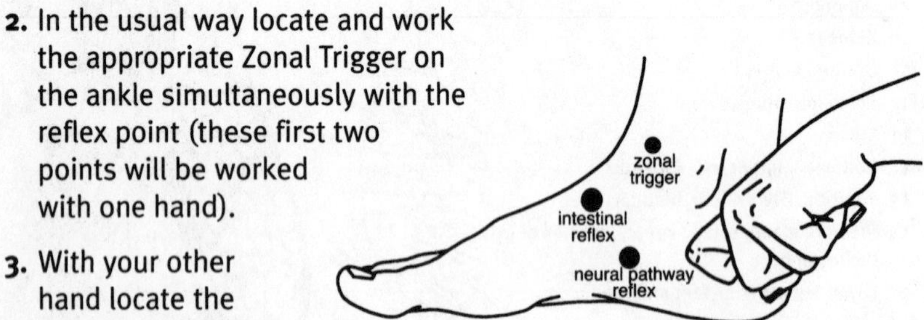

4. Briefly work all three reflexes at once and hold for a maximum of thirty seconds.
5. Repeat on the other foot.

Metatarsal Pressure on the cervical and spinal reflexes

The metatarsal bones are the longest bones in the feet, with the toes attached at one end and the collection of bones that make up the heel and ankle at the other. This technique takes pressure on the standing foot one stage further, as only the ball of the foot is placed on the ground so that the instep is arched. The extra pressure placed on the spinal reflexes appears to give more energy or stimulation to the appropriate reflexes, whether on the spine or other parts of the foot. It is particularly useful for helping neck, shoulder and back problems. Working the foot in this manner enables the reflexologist also to briefly access many of the reflexes on the sole, as long as the sensitive and taut tendon, between zone one and two, is totally avoided. Metatarsal Pressure is also an excellent form of self-help. The neural pathway reflexes can be stimulated with knuckles in this position.

Metatarsal Pressure can be substituted for working the normal spinal reflexes on the standing foot if required, followed by SR and ZT which can be applied in the usual manner.

Method

1. The client places one foot firmly on the ground and then lifts the arch of the other foot so he or she is pressing down on the ball of the foot in a stepping position.
2. Using the knuckle of your forefinger, or the side of your thumb, press firmly along the spinal reflexes starting from the axle/axis reflex on the big toe. This will usually feel very tender when you work a weak reflex.
3. Gently support the bent foot by placing your hand underneath on the sole and continue to work down the length of the spinal reflexes to the heel. This technique appears to allow even deeper access to the vertebrae reflexes. Always work both feet to balance.

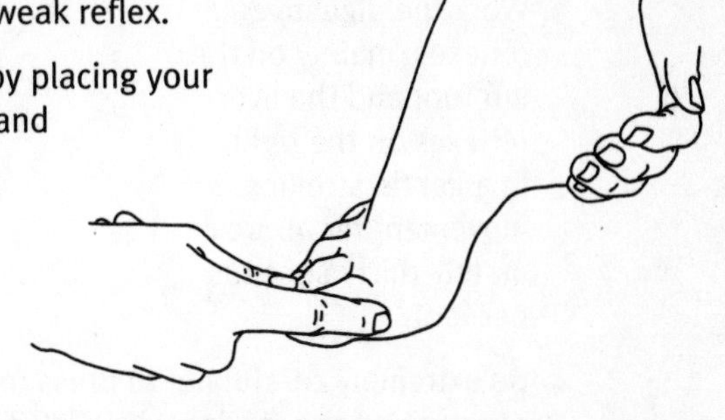

Case study

When one of my VRT tutors was on holiday she developed painful lower backache on the first day and was unable to lie down or walk for long without discomfort. She began using Metatarsal Pressure techniques on herself and almost immediately experienced relief. It was so comforting and effective to work the lower lumbar reflexes in this way that whenever her back began to ache she would stop, place her arched foot on a low wall or stair and work the reflexes for a few minutes. Within a few days the problem had cleared up completely.

Plantar Stepping

This is a useful technique if the practitioner wants greater access to the abdominal organs on the sole and it is particularly helpful for digestive problems. The aim is to slope the foot so that it is not under strain but is still weight-bearing, and so that some of the reflexes on the sole can be accessed at the same time.

Method

1. The sole of one foot is lifted off the ground (approximately 45 degrees), with pressure firmly applied on the supporting ball of the foot.
2. Place your four fingers on the sole while supporting the top of the foot with the thumb in a pinching movement on the outside or lateral edge of the foot.
3. Work the digestive reflexes, mainly on the left foot and the liver reflexes on the right, in a gentle stroking movement for approximately thirty seconds per foot.

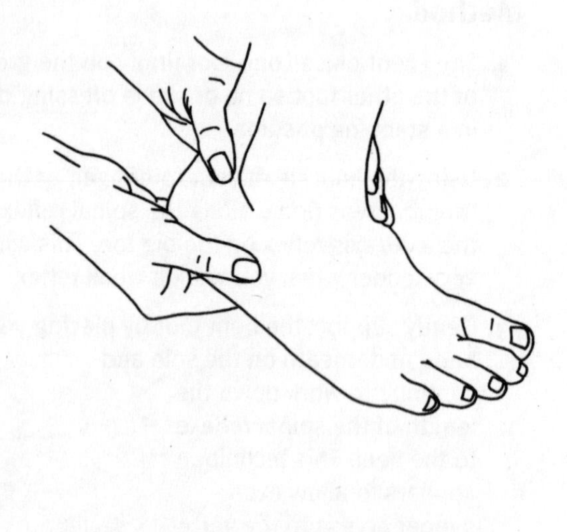

4. Be extremely careful not to press too firmly. It is essential to avoid pressure on the tendon which is situated on the inner side of the sole on each foot. The tendons, situated in zone one, are sensitive and vulnerable and should never be pressed when the foot is at a weight-bearing angle. The positive results obtained seem to depend not on pressure but on the angle of the foot, which appears to make deeper abdominal reflexes more accessible. Do not try and access the reflexes on the inside or medial side of the foot with this technique.

Knuckle Dusting

Knuckle Dusting is an unusual method of treating the body generally by making sweeping movements with the knuckles on the top of a standing foot. It appears to have a stimulating effect on the central nervous system, possibly by triggering a response from the nerve reflexes that spread out from the spinal cord reflexes to the various organs. This is an extremely powerful technique and should be limited to about fifteen or twenty seconds per foot. It appears to be very helpful for conditions as diverse as asthma, neck and shoulder problems and depression, and can be followed by the Palming technique (see p. 144).

The general outcome is an invigorating effect on the body and it may cause a momentary feeling of light-headedness, so ensure that there is always a table or chair available for support. Specific reflexes can be worked several times briefly, using an individual knuckle.

The toes are particularly sensitive to this treatment and sinus problems, headaches/tension and ear/eye problems respond well, as do sluggish digestive systems.

'My ten-year-old son still wets his bed from time to time, but my doctor says he will grow out of it. Would VRT help?'

In children, the cause is often psychological. Reflexology will help relax him, especially if you apply Diaphragm Rocking after five minutes of Basic VRT at bedtime. Work the bladder and lumbar spine synergistically, linking the brain reflexes with the Zonal Triggers. Apply Knuckle Dusting and Palming before finishing with the pituitary pinch.

Method

1. Make your hand into a fist with the thumb tucked inside.
2. Place your fist downwards on to the standing foot (or hand) and flick your wrist so that the second finger joints and knuckles touch and skim the foot (or hand) in a rolling, repetitive and twisting movement.
3. This technique should be lightly administered as it can be a little painful, even with a light touch.

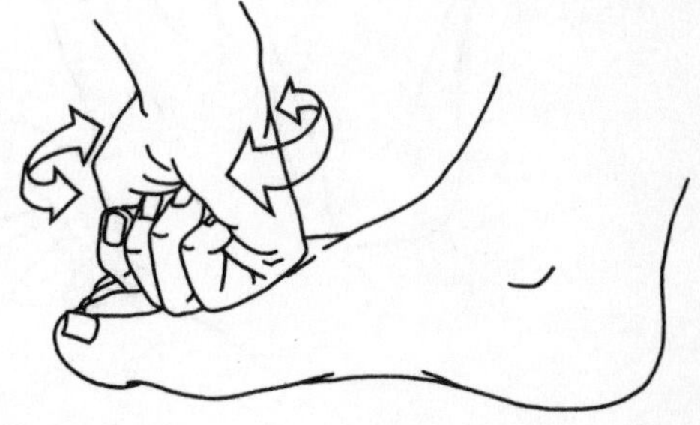

Palming

This is a gentle technique which uses the heel of the hand on the top of the standing foot not to massage but to apply firm pressure in a specific sweeping/twisting movement over the dorsal reflexes, and it can be practised for thirty to forty seconds on each foot. Palming can stimulate the reflexes, but also has a very calming and balancing effect on the body, unlike Knuckle Dusting which is highly stimulating. These two methods work well together as Knuckle Dusting appears to help the body make radical changes to its present condition, such as mild depression or asthma, almost immediately, whereas Palming appears to calm and centre the body and helps it to adjust at a more profound level after these changes have occurred. Palming is not easy, or as effective, to administer on the reclining feet, but it can be attempted by supporting the foot on the sole with the palm of your hand and pressing against it firmly while you treat the top of the foot with the other hand.

Method

1. Place your hand over the standing foot and tilt your wrist approximately 45 degrees so that your fingers are pointing upwards.
2. Use the heel of your palm, just above the wrist, to make a short rolling motion over the entire top of the foot aided by a twisting movement of the wrist.
3. When you touch sensitive reflexes work them by twisting the lateral, or outer, base of the palm over a specific area several times.

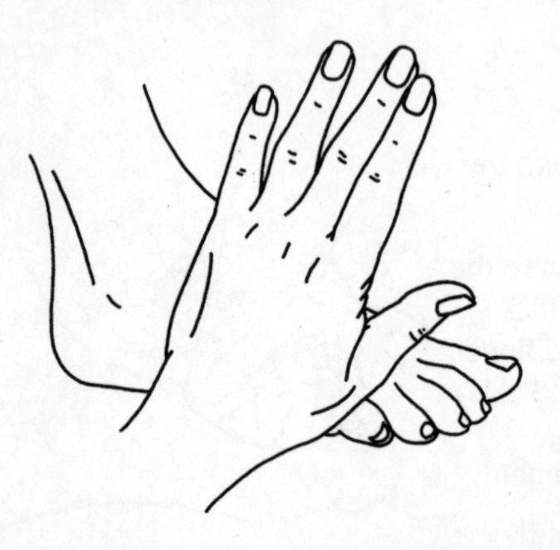

Sample VRT treatments using some advanced techniques

The sequences described below can be used either side of a VRT treatment, but not both.

General method

At the start of a treatment:

1. Work swiftly over the standing feet for a total of about two minutes gently pressing and working the pelvic/ankle reflexes, the spinal reflexes and the toes.
2. Note any tender points on the top of the foot and work gently, followed by some brief Palming.
3. Work the feet with conventional reflexology, using Diaphragm Rocking and Lymphatic Stimulation midway through the session.

At the completion of a treatment:

What you do now depends on the condition that needs attention. Below are two examples: irritable bowel and asthma.

Irritable bowel

Begin by giving a quick two-minute Basic VRT treatment following the Step-by-Step Instructions at the end of Chapter 5 and insert the following advanced techniques:

- After 4.a the 'banana' movement, use Plantar Stepping techniques. Work the bowel/colon reflexes gently on both feet, avoiding the tendon on the inside (zone one) of the sole.
- After 4.b and c, spinal reflexes, stimulate the neural pathway reflexes for the bowel by pressing the L1 reflex with your knuckles or side of the thumb. Work roughly in the area indicated in the chart in this chapter and you should be guided to the right spot by a pinprick sensation on a tender reflex.
- While holding this reflex find the Zonal Trigger on the ankle and press the two points simultaneously.
- Work three reflexes together. If you have found one painful reflex on the colon, press it with your forefinger while holding the ZT reflex with your thumb. With your other hand locate and press L1 on the spinal reflex with your knuckle so that you are holding three points simultaneously for approximately thirty seconds.

- After no. 7, lymphatic reflexes, use Knuckle Dusting on both feet to stimulate the digestive and excretory systems.
- To soothe the feet perform a Palming action with the heel of your hand over the top of the foot for about thirty seconds.
- Continue to complete the Basic VRT treatment.

Asthma

Begin to give a Basic VRT treatment following the Step-by-Step Instructions at the end of Chapter 5 and insert the following advanced techniques:

- After no. 4, spinal reflexes. Use your knuckle, or side of the thumb, to apply Metatarsal Pressure on the cervical/spinal reflexes to the ball of the foot so that the T3 reflex (respiratory system) is stimulated – it may feel very tender on both feet.
- After no. 7, lymphatic reflexes, which you would work three times, use Knuckle Dusting and Palming on the metatarsal (chest reflex) area on the top of the foot.
- After no. 10, metatarsals, when the whole foot has been worked stimulate the adrenal points on both feet simultaneously for thirty seconds.
- No. 13, the pituitary pinch – conclude by holding for forty-five rather than thirty seconds.

Conventional reflexology treatment for asthma

With asthma it can be very beneficial to perform Diaphragm Rocking for longer (two to three minutes), as it relaxes the ribcage/diaphragm and can ease congested lungs. Extend Lymphatic Stimulation by a minute per foot. Work several Zonal Triggers relating the chest, lungs, ileocecal valve and adrenals in the reclining position, as the reactions are less powerful.

Experiment in your approach to using all the techniques relating to VRT

- Always start with the ankles and Zonal Trigger area, followed by the spinal reflexes. You can choose to give the Basic VRT treatment twice (two bursts of three to four minutes) at the beginning and end of a session.
- You can also treat gently for only one or two minutes with no conventional reflexology, and still get results.
- Experiment with the introduction of advanced techniques approximately in the middle of the VRT session, and gradually you will become quicker at discerning which is most appropriate for a certain condition.

Reminder

- Treat chronic conditions two to three times a week to let the body heal itself.
- Acute conditions can be treated once or twice daily.
- Self-help techniques can be used at least twice daily for a minute or two for chronic conditions and several times daily for acute ailments.
- Advanced techniques do not have to be used during every treatment, but it is recommended that one or two are used in each session to consolidate VRT and reflexology.

Key points to remember

- **Advanced techniques enhance treatments but are an optional addition to Basic VRT.**
- **Do not apply advanced techniques without at least working the ankles and the spinal reflexes first with VRT.**
- **The neural pathway reflexes are worked much more effectively when the knuckles or the edge of the thumb are used.**
- **Do not work the hand reflex synergistically when selecting the most tender neural pathway reflex. Instead work the standard dorsal reflex and the Zonal Trigger with the neural pathway reflex on the spine, i.e. all three reflexes are on the feet.**
- **Always use Metatarsal Pressure if there are neck and shoulder problems.**
- **Plantar Stepping is useful for working part of the sole of the foot, but avoid pressure on the tendons.**
- **Knuckle Dusting – work quickly and cover the entire foot with swift twisting movements. Check that the client is holding on to a chair and that the reflexes are not too tender.**
- **Palming – use the edge of the heel of your palm so that you can work smaller areas of the foot, focusing on clusters of reflexes.**
- **Experiment with VRT treatments for specific ailments, and try different permutations using advanced techniques.**
- **Remember to use all the advanced techniques on the hands when working them in a weight-bearing position.**

VRT self-help techniques

REFLEXOLOGY IS ONE OF THE MORE ACCOMMODATING THERAPIES WHEN IT COMES to self-help techniques, and with VRT there is also a heightened sense of awareness and effectiveness. Osteopaths, aromatherapists and acupuncturists, for example, are often unable to minister to their own needs and rely on colleagues to treat them. But reflexologists can easily access their own hands and feet and work them very effectively. However, qualified reflexologists often comment that while they obtain reasonable results on themselves they cannot tune into their own needs or feel much sensitivity. It becomes mechanical, rather than intuitive, which is often the case when there is no exchange of energy between two people. Vertical Reflex Therapy and Synergistic Reflexology enable us to treat ourselves more effectively in terms of both results and the greater degree of information we receive from our bodies as we work on our feet.

Everyone who can should look after themselves and take responsibility for their own needs. Self-help VRT is as useful when we are seriously ill as when we just have a cold. We all need to help stimulate the body to heal itself, to bring about better health and to prevent minor health problems becoming major illnesses. The ideal formula is to have regular professional reflexology treatments and in between to give yourself a brief self-help treatment as part of a regular maintenance programme.

'My fourteen-year-old daughter has very painful, heavy periods. Can VRT help?'

VRT is extremely helpful for all sorts of menstrual problems, even long-term ones. Young girls especially can benefit from VRT – while their bodies are still growing it is a good idea to stimulate the hormonal system to regulate their periods. Two or three minutes of self-help VRT twice a day could be all that your daughter needs.

In your own self-help practice sessions I suggest you press firmly enough to feel slight discomfort in areas you know to be sensitive. For example, if you suffer from neck problems then the base and medial side of the thumb and big toe will feel tender. Press firmly as you work that area, but if it actually becomes too painful back off and work more lightly. It is a good exercise to use VRT on yourself because you will become much more aware of the different levels of discomfort when the feet or hands are weight-bearing than if you were using conventional self-help reflexology.

The advantage of self-help Hand Reflexology is that it can be applied in the workplace or on social occasions without attracting too much attention to oneself. However, if the benefits of Self-help VRT outweigh being the object of curiosity for you, be bold and work on your feet whenever the need arises!

These VRT skills will become invaluable as first aid at home, at work or travelling. You will be able to react quickly if you fall and injure yourself or perhaps feel a stomach ache or sore throat coming on. Chronic problems can be alleviated by learning to work the appropriate reflexes for a few seconds whenever you feel discomfort. But generally the techniques in this chapter should become part of your general maintenance programme to keep in good health.

It is important to build up the self-help skills in a methodical way. So, even if you are a professional reflexologist, briefly treat a few reflex points on your feet in the conventional manner so that you can experience the contrasting improvement once you apply Synergistic Reflexology and VRT.

As with all VRT treatments it does not matter whether you start with the left or right foot. There is only one important rule with any form of Synergistic Reflexology, and that is that the right hand works the right foot and the left hand works the left foot. This is to enable the energy from the stimulated hand and foot reflexes to flow through the same zone on the same side of the body.

'The menopause is giving me severe hot flushes, bloating and a generally "spaced out" feeling. Self-help VRT to my toes and ankles is not achieving much. What else can I do?'

To balance the entire body, especially the endocrine system, many women do the full but brief VRT treatment described on pp. 155–7 morning and night. Try working particularly round the thyroid and pituitary reflexes on the big toes, and find the Zonal Trigger associated with both. Also locate the ZT on the wrist and then, when you have a hot flush, apply standard hand reflexology if you are unable to use VRT on your hands and feet. Although it is preferable to press the ZT and reflexes simultaneously, you can work the pituitary and thyroid reflexes on the thumbs first and then press the ZTs on the wrists to help regulate the body's thermostat. Work the ovary and ovary helper reflexes firmly. Self-help VRT can be given twice daily or more. Weekly full VRT/reflexology treatments will be very beneficial until your hormonal system is regulated, after which you should have a maintenance treatment every four weeks.

The standard approach to self-help reflexology involves a reasonably agile person sitting down and placing one foot on their lap while working the reflexes. For years I have used this approach to give myself a good treatment and, if you find you are always too busy, why not treat your feet when you are a passenger on a long car journey? With Synergistic Reflexology I can now work my hand and foot at the same time! It is much easier than it sounds, and the illustrations in this chapter will indicate each step. For the most beneficial form of self-help VRT, stand and place your foot on a wooden chair or stool and work the top of the foot as you lean forward to exert more weight. If you are unable to reach your feet, or feel that you may overbalance, place your hand palm downwards in a weight-bearing position on a table and work the top of the hand.

A choice of four techniques

You can treat yourself with reflexology and VRT in any of the following ways: these techniques will come easily when the need arises

Conventional self-help:

Sit down and work your feet in the conventional manner by placing each foot on your lap as you work the reflexes.

Synergistic self-help:

Sit down and treat your feet as described immediately above. Next find up to three priority reflexes that need working. Your right hand works the reflex on your right foot while your left forefinger works your right hand. Follow the step-by-step instructions on pp. 152–4 and all will become clear immediately! You can even work a Zonal Trigger in this way.

Standing self-help VRT and synergistic reflexology:

Stand and place your foot on a chair. Work the hand and foot simultaneously as with synergistic self-help.

Self-help hand reflexology and VRT:

Place your hand firmly on a table palm downwards apply and basic VRT techniques to the dorsum of the hand.

Conventional self-help

Method

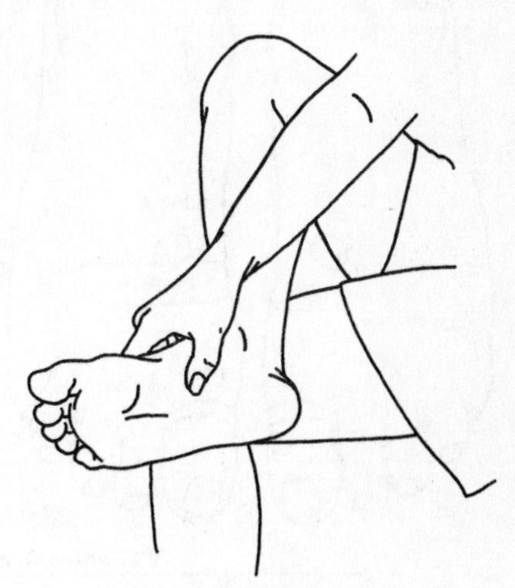

Self-help treatment – sitting

1. Sit comfortably in an upright or easy chair. A bed is not very suitable as your back will not be supported and you will be at the wrong angle. However, if you are ill in bed and can comfortably reach your feet, it is better than nothing.
2. Lift up one leg and place your foot across your other thigh so that you can grasp your foot firmly with both hands.
3. Work the foot by gently loosening it and pressing the reflexes, using the appropriate relaxation techniques shown in Chapter 4.
4. Using the guidelines in Chapter 5 or your skills as a reflexologist, work swiftly over the various systems of the body to stimulate it generally and practise a few relaxation techniques. Work each foot for between five and fifteen minutes, paying special attention to tender reflexes that can indicate an imbalance in the body. A tender reflex does not necessarily indicate major disease or a problem you didn't know you had, it can simply mean there is a slight imbalance that reflexology can help correct. In the long term, regular VRT and reflexology can help to balance the body and prevent health problems developing.
5. Finally, select the following reflexes and work them firmly on both feet:
   - Adrenal glands.
   - Neck.
   - Stomach.

These reflexes have been selected to give variety in this practice session because the adrenals are found on both feet, the stomach is found mainly on the left foot and the neck on the big toe. It is important to be conscious of the pressure and response you get from these three reflexes as you will now work the same three reflexes on the hands and feet synergistically and compare the sensations.

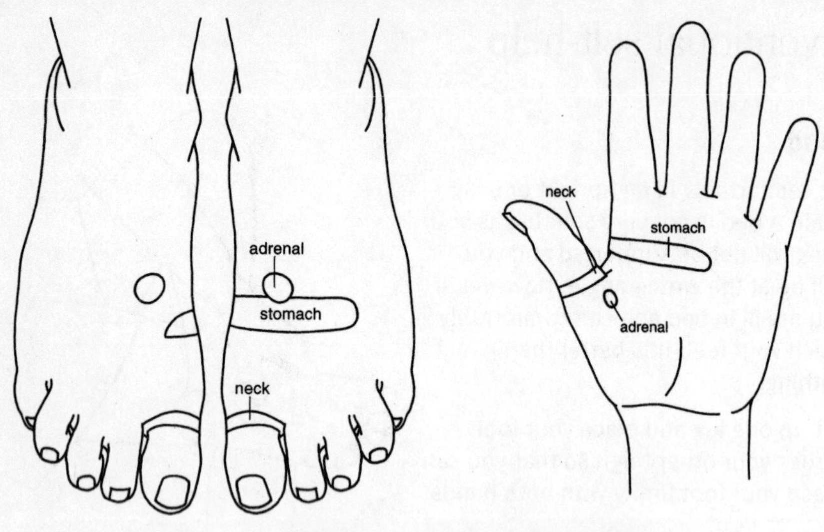

VRT adrenal, neck and stomach reflexes

Synergistic self-help

The aim of this exercise is to teach you to 'turn up the power' of the stimulated reflexes by working the hands and feet together. The powerful effect of two reflexes worked simultaneously can be experienced when you work on yourself. It is this aspect of the treatment that enables you not only to feel your own reflexes being worked more deeply but also to have a heightened sensitivity that usually only happens when someone else is working on your feet.

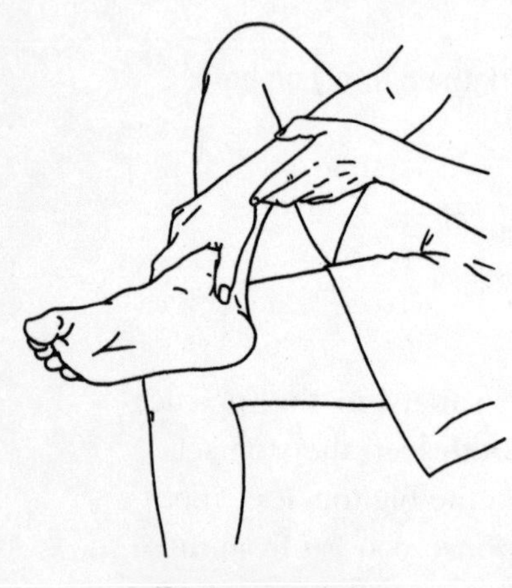
Self-help synergistic treatment – sitting

General method

1 Work and relax both feet as described for conventional self-help above. You can start with your left or right foot. During this brief ten-minute treatment identify up to three priority reflexes that require treatment, relating to the parts of your body that are imbalanced or malfunctioning in some way. These points could be as diverse as a neck reflex because your neck has just become stiff, the lung reflexes due to chronic asthma, or the uterus due to period pain. Minor ailments and chronic illnesses can both respond to Synergistic Reflexology.

2. Having worked both feet, return to work on the foot with which you started. Remember the rule: left hand/left foot, right hand/right foot.
3. The same three reflexes worked on with conventional self-help (see p. 151) will be used for this exercise, so that a contrast can be made between the sensations in the foot when two reflexes are worked simultaneously. The foot reflexes invariably become more tender and the hand reflexes, which can be less sensitive at first, sometimes throb or become warm.

You can start with either hand and foot, but I shall use the right each time for continuity. Afterwards, repeat the same procedures on the other hand and foot. The adrenal reflexes will be found in the same position on both feet. Different neck reflexes may feel sensitive as you will be working on both sides of the neck, so adjust the working of the hands and feet accordingly until you find a tender reflex. The stomach reflexes cover a larger part of the plantar (sole) on the left foot, so work carefully over this area to ensure that you have completely treated it.

Adrenal reflex

1. Sit down and place your right foot on your left thigh.
2. Locate the adrenal reflex on your right hand with your left forefinger and press firmly. It is easy to locate as it will feel slightly bruised in most cases. This is simply a sign of vitality, but if you are very stressed it could feel quite painful.
3. Maintain pressure on the hand adrenal reflex and move your right hand down to the adrenal point on the right sole and work it firmly with your thumb for about thirty seconds. If you find that your brain cannot cope with working both points at once, don't worry! Simply press the reflex on your hand firmly while you work into the adrenal point on the palm of your hand.

'I suffer from recurrent cystitis. Can VRT help?'

Yes, especially when used in conjunction with other remedies such as cranberry capsules. It is particularly helpful at the onset of an attack, when the adrenals, bladder and urethra reflexes should be worked firmly in the weight-bearing position on the feet two or three times a day and every hour or so on the hands. Self-help Metatarsal Pressure is particularly useful, and you can firmly work the lower lumbar spine and urinary system at the same time. Remember also to be very careful about personal hygiene, especially before and after sex, and to drink plenty of water at all times.

Neck reflex

1. Move straight on to the neck reflex on the same foot. Remember that you are trying to locate the most tender reflex in a certain area, so work your thumb and fingers very precisely in case you miss it.
2. Before I start treating a client's neck I usually get them to loosen up their neck reflexes in a way that is very effective in preparing the neck reflexes, but cannot be considered to be pure reflexology! You can use this same technique on yourself now. Clench your left fingers round your right thumb and hold it firmly. Twist your right hand backwards and forwards while your right thumb remains static and gripped tightly. Repeat on the other hand.
3. Pinch round the base of your right thumb with your left thumb and finger and try to locate a tender neck reflex. Most people hold some tension in their neck, and you may find that the most sensitive point is on the medial (inside) of the thumb towards the nail. This would indicate a possible tension in one of the cervical vertebrae.
4. Maintain pressure on the hand neck reflex and move your right hand down to the neck point on the right big toe (see p. 152). Work the corresponding point with your left thumb or forefinger for about thirty seconds. This could be round the base of the toe or on the medial or even lateral side. Press the hand reflex firmly if you are unable to rotate two points at once.

Stomach reflex

1. Most of our stomach is positioned on the left of our body, so naturally the stomach reflex is located on the left foot except for a small reflex on the right foot and hand on the medial edge (see p. 152).
2. Locate the stomach reflex on your left hand with your right forefinger, not thumb, and work this small area firmly.
3. Maintain the pressure on the hand stomach reflex as you move your left hand down to the stomach reflex on the left sole of your foot and work the corresponding point with your right thumb. Press the hand reflex firmly if you are unable to work the two reflexes at once.

Case study

Tara, a highly intelligent nine-year-old, was medically declared to be suffering from a mystery illness. She had been incredibly thin and debilitated for months, had constantly aching joints, and had to be wheeled to school when she was well enough to attend. She had attacks of violent diarrhoea several times a week. A large lump of thickened tissue had formed on the dorsum of each hand under the skin, and the doctors were deciding whether to surgically remove them although they were not sure what had caused them. She had been seen by numerous consultants who had performed many tests. It later turned out that she had a complex form of lupus, an inflammatory disease.

I gently used weight-bearing techniques on the dorsal reflexes (on the top of her feet) and found they were extremely tender. I suggested she took some basic nutritional supplements and avoided certain foods, and taught her various self-help techniques. This was a very holistic approach that incorporated reflexology, VRT, nutritional advice and various types of medication much later from her doctors. She was amazingly positive and interested in helping herself, and her parents were very supportive.

One of the first improvements was that the strange lumps on her hands began to shrink. Within weeks her diarrhoea attacks had abated and her joints were aching less. She continued to work on herself with reflexology to top up my treatments. Within three months she was able to run in a race at her school sports day and go on shopping trips with her mother. She was delighted to be able to walk to school again.

Standing self-help VRT and Synergistic Reflexology

The basic requirement is that you are physically able to stand without support and can place your foot on a wooden stool, chair or stair. A padded or upholstered chair is not firm enough but will do if nothing else is available. I have also seen very flexible people bend, touch their toes and apply a VRT treatment with both their feet on the floor!

Your body is much more receptive to reflexology in a standing position, so the following sequence of techniques is the ultimate in your self-help programme. As you become more familiar with the hand reflexes you will easily adapt these basic techniques to suit your individual needs. The only VRT techniques that do not translate to

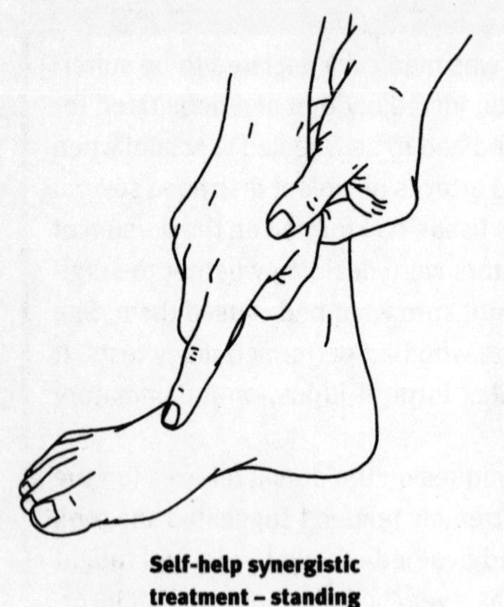

Self-help synergistic treatment – standing

self-help on the feet are Diaphragm Rocking and Lymphatic Stimulation. Both can be used on the hands with a moderate degree of success (see p. 164).

To experience the full VRT treatment you can follow the instructions from the Basic Instructions at the end of Chapter 5 and firmly apply to yourself the sequence of techniques that you have already learnt to apply to others. There is one important difference when treating yourself: you do not have to keep changing feet, as your own energy seems to keep you in balance. So complete the entire treatment on one foot before starting on the other.

You can use the following shortened version to relax and loosen up after a busy day and concentrate on two synergistic points that are appropriate to your particular needs, for example, the shoulder and kidney, plus one priority Zonal Trigger, uterus/prostate. If you are fortunate enough to be perfectly fit, work the neck, shoulders and adrenals as a general tonic.

Method for general VRT self-help treatment

As before, I have always started with the right hand and foot just for continuity. When you have finished, repeat the procedures on the left foot and hand.

1. Place your right foot on a chair and lean slightly forward so that it is bearing as much of your weight as possible without tilting you forward.

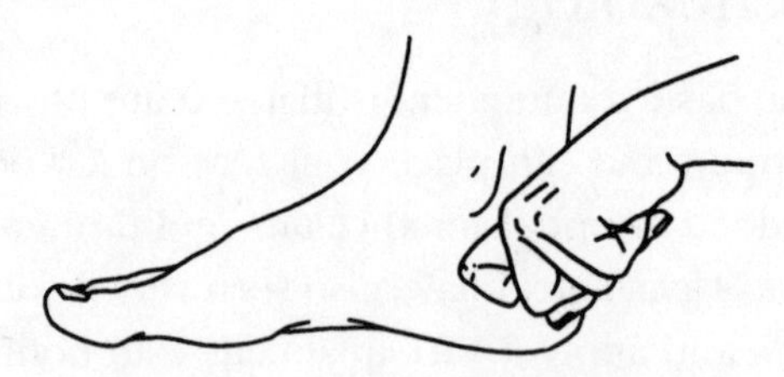

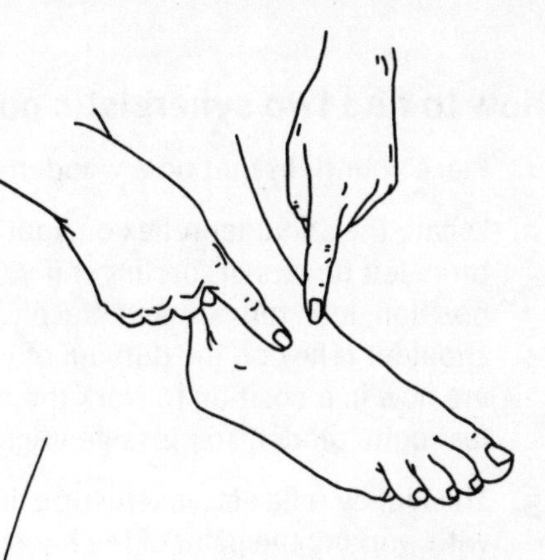

2. Using both hands, work swiftly round the ankles and the pelvic/hip reflexes using fingers, thumbs and knuckles.

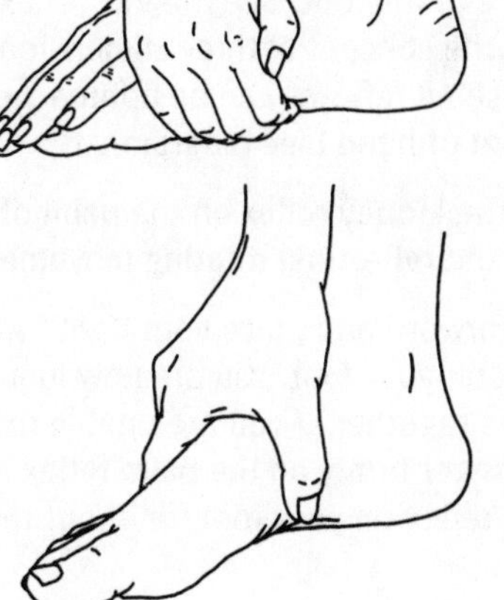

3. Slip your fingers under the arch of your foot and pull on the spinal reflexes to relax the lower back. This physically stretches the back as well as stimulating the appropriate reflexes.

4. Press spinal reflexes from toe to heel with thumb. Firmly tap up and down the inside (medial) of the foot along the spinal reflexes. Support the top of your foot firmly with the other hand.

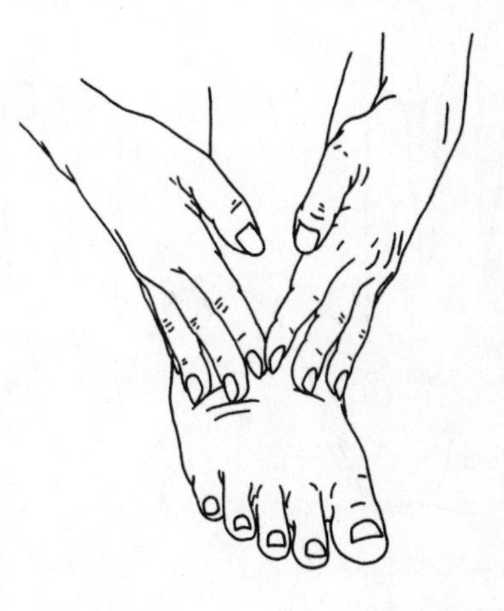

5. Using the fingertips of both hands, work down the dorsum of the foot from the ankles to the toes. Make the fingers 'caterpillar' walk in tiny bites so that the entire top of the foot, and therefore all the main organs, are stimulated.

6. Press firmly on the toes as they contain all the head, neck, ear, eye and nose reflexes, plus some of the main endocrine glands such as the pituitary, thyroid and pineal. Some reflexologists also refer, as part of their treatment, to the basic acupuncture meridian points that begin in the toes. If you firmly work the toes you will certainly be stimulating acupressure points as well, although there is considerable debate among reflexologists whether these two therapies overlap.

How to find two synergistic points when self-treating

1. Place your right foot on a wooden chair or stool.
2. Locate the shoulder reflex on your right hand and work it with your three left fingers or forefinger if you find it easier. Maintaining this position, lean forward and place your three right fingers on the shoulder reflex on the dorsum of your right foot (see diagram). You are now in a position to work the reflexes together. They will probably feel quite tender, so press gently but firmly for thirty seconds.
3. The kidney reflex is a useful practice example as it familiarises you with working the palm of the hand, which is easily accessed, and the top of the foot. The dorsal reflexes, including the kidneys on the top of the foot, are a new approach to reflexes because they are usually accessed from the plantar or sole of the foot. See the VRT reflexology plantar chart on p. 72. With VRT the concept of three-dimensional zones is developed, so that the same reflexes can be approached from the top or bottom of the foot or hand (see diagram).
4. With your left forefinger locate the kidney reflex on the palm of your right hand, and press and work the reflex in a rotating movement.
5. Maintaining this position, lean forward and place your right forefinger on the right dorsal kidney reflex on your foot. You are now in a position to work the two reflexes together. If you are unable to rotate both points at once, hold your finger firmly on the palm reflex and rotate and stimulate the kidney reflex on your foot for about thirty seconds.

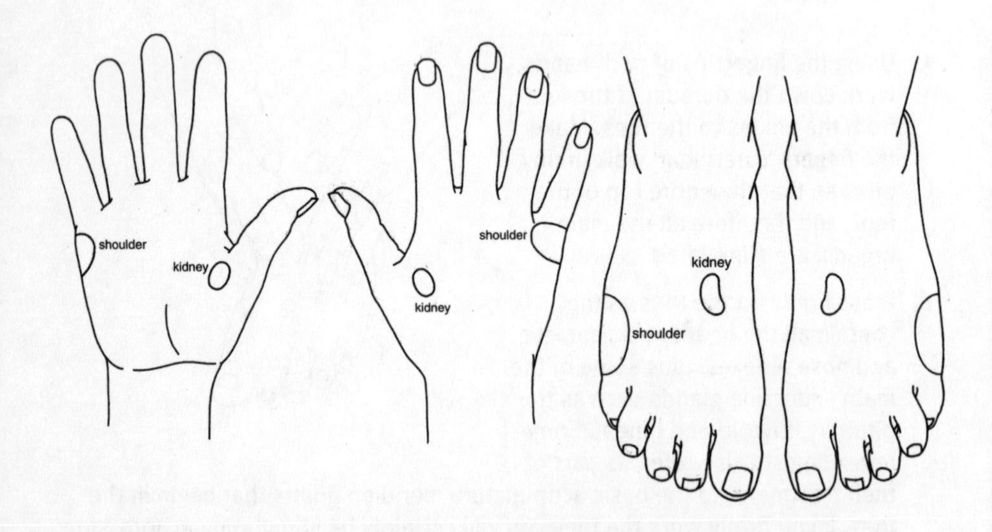

Position of kidney and shoulder reflexes on the palm, back of hand and feet.

Finally, find one priority Zonal Trigger while standing

The uterus/prostate reflex has been selected as the three-point Zonal Trigger because it provides good practise in accessing the reflexes on the medial side of the hands and feet. The Zonal Triggers are, as explained in Chapter 7, an extremely powerful set of ankle reflexes that should be used with care when the feet are in a standing position as they channel extra healing energy to the part of the body that needs it most at that time. Hence only one reflex should be worked in this manner during any particular treatment. The body is galvanised into an extra surge of energy/rebalancing when a Zonal Trigger is pressed. If that energy is directed to more than one part of the body during a treatment it could cause the body to over-react and a temporary healing crisis could occur.

1. Locate the uterus/prostate reflex on the medial or inside of the right ankle (see p. 160) with your right thumb and work it gently for a few seconds. This pressure signals that you have made a connection with a certain reflex and now want to find the corresponding Zonal Trigger on the ankle. You can now take your finger off the reflex.
2. To locate the Zonal Trigger use your left forefinger or right thumb, and begin pressing along the ZT band which is situated about 5mm above the medial right ankle bone. A Zonal Trigger is usually, but not always, situated in the same zone as the reflex being worked. In this particular case it would be zone one.
3. When you reach the correct Zonal Trigger there is often a sharp pin-prick sensation that indicates the correct location. If one is not immediately apparent, continue to move round towards the outer ankles. On the rare occasion when a trigger point is not located anywhere in the band, return to the zone in which the reflex is situated and work that zone. With Zonal Triggers it is important that you are guided more by a slightly painful sensation, which indicates you have hit the right spot, than the location of the zone in relation to the reflex. If you hit a tender point move past it for a few centimetres to check you have hit the most tender spot.
4. You are now ready to work the three reflexes at once. While you are practising, it is useful to work slowly to see if you can detect a warmth in the reflex or organ being treated as you increase the energy by introducing the reflexes one by one. VRT achieves results when there is no sensation at all, but it is helpful to be aware of the possible sensations.

Method

1. Locate the uterus/prostate reflex on your right foot using your right thumb. Remember to lean your leg well forward on the chair for maximum weight-bearing pressure.
2. Place your right forefinger on the Zonal Trigger you have previously located. Your right thumb and forefinger are splayed apart so they touch the two points at the same time.
3. Bring your left hand down to your right hand, which is working the foot, and locate with your left forefinger the uterus/prostate point on the medial side of the right hand at wrist level.
4. Work all three points together. You will probably find it easier to work the ankle and wrist reflexes in a slightly rotating movement and just keep your forefinger positioned on the Zonal Trigger. Work the reflexes for about thirty seconds, then repeat on the other foot.

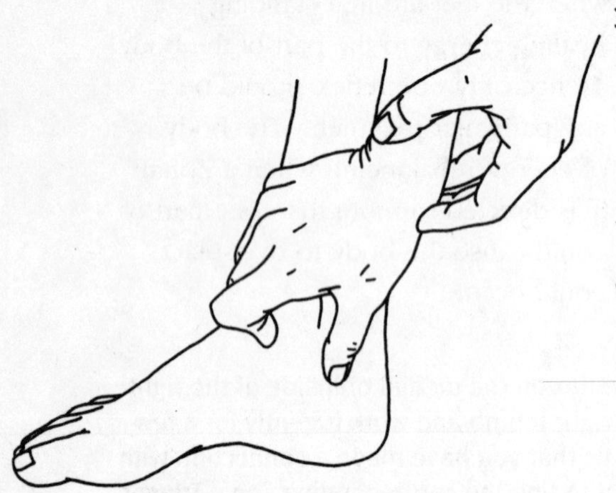

Working three reflexes at once including the Zonal Trigger

Even if you have a one-sided problem, such as a stiff shoulder, the reflexes on the other foot should be worked as well to balance the body. It is always especially helpful in orthopaedic cases because the body will often be unbalanced due to uneven posture or referred pain.

Once you have mastered the basic concept of treating yourself using the various VRT techniques you will be able to tailor brief treatments to your immediate needs. The Zonal Triggers are profound healing tools for your repertoire, and a short time spent practising them will reap numerous long-term benefits for you and those you treat.

Case study

Two years ago I managed to fall two metres into our boat from the quayside, and it would probably have been a lot less painful if I had hit the water! Apart from being very embarrassed I was badly shaken, having hit my head, back and shoulders on the controls and seating. My young daughter suggested VRT, which was just as well as I was not thinking straight. I placed my foot on the seat and gingerly began some self-help VRT, concentrating on the back and neck synergistically and the Zonal Triggers for the shoulder. I could feel my shoulder become warm almost immediately. I then stood up and asked her to work my feet as I stood. It was really just a rather amateurish attempt to press the entire dorsum quickly, with me giving the instructions. After two or three minutes I began to feel clicks, tingling and warmth in various parts of my body as it began to relax and recover. Over the years, many people have told me they could feel their body adjusting and correcting itself as I worked on their feet. The boating accident allowed me to experience this sensation for myself.

Self-help hand reflexology and VRT

There are many occasions when people could treat themselves with VRT but do not want to draw attention to themselves by placing their foot on a chair and performing in public. It is, however, very easy and discreet to place your hand firmly on a table or hard surface and work the reflexes with your other hand. You can even select a Zonal Trigger, as well as working a reflex on the top of the hand. This way you reach the same reflexes that you find on the palm but, like VRT on the feet, they are approached from above.

If you have a painful shoulder or stomach ache, for example, you can give yourself VRT on your feet morning and evening, including three points using the Zonal Triggers and Synergistic Reflexology. During the day you can top up the treatment on your hands.

To offer a variety of practice moves we shall work the sinus reflexes on the dorsum; the breast reflexes, which are always found on the lateral top of the hands, and the ovary/testes and helper ovary/testes reflexes.

Method for general hand VRT

1. Stand and place your flattened palm firmly on a table with your arm straight, leaning on it slightly to take some of your weight. Once weight-bearing, the reflexes will become more responsive in the same way as with standard VRT. Splay your fingers out slightly.
2. Work the entire hand first by following the basic VRT Hand Crib Sheet at the end of Chapter 9.
3. You may have to adjust your angles slightly, but the aim is to cover the entire hand with tiny pressure impulses to stimulate the entire body quickly. Remember to work down the arms and across the wrist to stimulate the lymphatic reflexes and boost your immune system.
4. Repeat the treatment on the other hand, allowing up to two minutes per hand. As with foot VRT, select two synergistic points and one priority Zonal Trigger.

Practice moves using sinus, breast, ovary/testes reflexes

The sinus reflexes

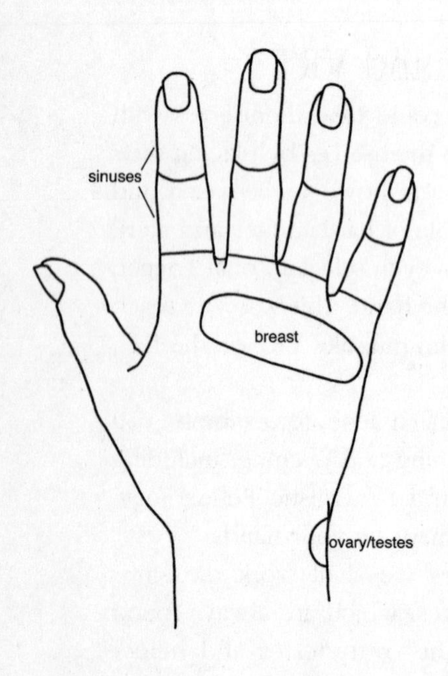

Position of the sinus, ovary/testes and breast reflexes on the hand

1. The sinus reflexes are situated on all the fingers, with some on the thumb. Although they are traditionally shown on the fingertips, I get a better response when I work each of the entire fingers as the ear reflexes at the base of the fingers are also worked at the same time. Many chronic sinus conditions affect the ears as well as the nasal passages.
2. Begin by working on your right forefinger by pinching the sides of it with your left forefinger and thumb. Start at the base of the finger and pinch up to the nail. Make two passes up the finger and then gently press and rotate your forefinger down from the nail, covering the entire length of your finger once.
3. Move on to your next finger, and repeat the process until all four fingers and the thumb have been worked.
4. Repeat the process on the other hand.

The breast reflexes

1. These are situated on the dorsum of the hands in conventional reflexology, and VRT charts and reflexes reflect the conventional anatomical position in the body. Ensure that you work the entire breast area with your fingertips, working into the reflexes with a firm touch and a rotating movement.
2. Return to rework any area that feels granular or tender to the touch. By working the entire breast area regularly you can assist lymph drainage generally, which is important for both men and women.
3. Repeat the process on the left hand.

The ovary/testes reflexes

These are conventionally situated on the lateral side of the hand at the wrist line (on the edge of the hand), see diagram – Conventional and Hand Reflexes. In VRT the helper ovary/testes reflex is situated in the middle of the palm about 5cm above the wrist in what I feel is a more anatomically correct position. This reflex can also be accessed via the dorsum and links with the helper ovary/testes foot reflex at mid-ankle. I work both helper and conventional reflexes to ensure that all avenues of stimulation are covered. Hand VRT allows you to access both reflexes easily.

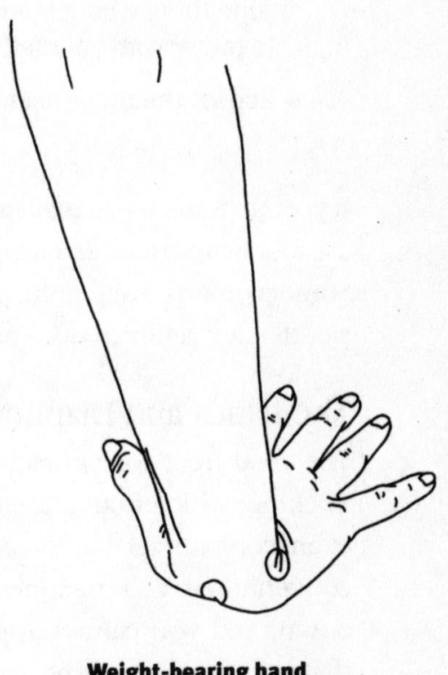

Weight-bearing hand with two ovary/testes reflexes

1. Press the ovary/testes point with your left thumb on your right hand and rotate firmly for about 15 seconds and repeat the pressure on the helper ovary/testes reflex as well.
2. Repeat the process on the left hand.

3. Ensure that your hand is firmly pressed on to the table at all times and is bearing as much of your weight as is comfortable. If this is the 'priority' reflex to be worked, you can locate the Zonal Trigger on the middle of the wrist band on the dorsum of your hand in the following way:
   - Press the right helper ovary/testes reflex – on the middle of the heel of your palm – with your left index finger in a rotating movement.
   - Using your left thumb or index finger in tiny 'bites' round the wrist band until you feel a sharp pinprick sensation. It will probably be located in the same zone as the helper ovary/testes reflex in zone three.
   - If you cannot feel the pinprick anywhere on the wrist band return to zone three where the reflex is situated and work the two points together with your left thumb and forefinger for about 30 seconds.
   - Repeat the process on the other hand.

If you are female you may find that the ovary/testes reflexes on one hand are much more tender than the other depending on your menstrual cycle. Some women have painful periods every other month and a left- or right-sided ovary reflex may be particularly tender during that cycle.

The hands and Diaphragm Rocking

The final treat for yourself when working your hands is Diaphragm Rocking, which is an extremely helpful aid to sleep and relaxation and even combats jet lag. It is normally used in the middle to end of a conventional/VRT treatment when the person being treated is lying down, and you cannot apply it to your own feet with any degree of rhythm or success. The hands certainly come a poor second to the calming, relaxing sensation of someone rocking your feet and pumping energy to the area most in need in your body. But try the following technique next time you have insomnia or are stressed. If you have a particular health problem and have treated your hands or feet with VRT, conclude with some Diaphragm Hand Rocking.

1. Hold your right hand in front of you with your elbow to your side and the palm facing you. Place your left thumb on the solar plexus reflex and press firmly.
2. Slightly lift your fingers up and over the thumb which is resting at the top of the third metacarpal, and bend them towards you.

3. Hold your thumb still and let your hand do the work by gently rocking your fingers forward and backward in a rhythmic movement. Once you feel relaxed enough stop thinking about each rocking movement, let the hand take over as it rocks backward and forward for a minute or two.
4. Repeat the process on the left hand.

This is a simple but profoundly effective technique that can be used on its own or to enhance one of the treatments described in this chapter.

Enhancing regular reflexology with self-help treatments

Therapists often attend my courses and say how delighted they are to receive a reflexology treatment during the final practical session as it is the first one they have had in months! We should all practise what we preach, and be considerate to our bodies by giving them regular attention with self-help VRT and treatments from other reflexologists. Once you are on the receiving end of a treatment you can appreciate the quality of time to be still, to learn from the person treating you and affirm your own approach to reflexology.

If you are new to reflexology or thinking about making it your career, experiment by having treatments from a few reflexologists and find out who and what suits you. There are many competent schools of reflexology which all teach in a slightly different way. You may find that you prefer a firm pressure to a very light touch. Both ways can be very effective, and I personally prefer to use a pressure that is firm enough to give some authority to my work without causing undue pain or discomfort. You do not want a client or friend to leave limping because you have been too rough or complaining that they had just had their feet tickled! In the Far East, some reflexologists work very quickly and painfully with little rounded sticks and their patients hobble away, confident they will feel much better within hours. It is extremely unwise to use sticks on the feet without proper training, so do not be tempted to try.

VRT can also accelerate the healing processes, but with little pain or few side-effects. The more you experience the wonderful scope of

Case study

Geoff was a thirty-nine-year-old business man who suffered from indigestion, especially if he drank alcohol and ate a rich meal at lunchtime. Years previously I had taught him gently to press the stomach reflex on his left hand after a large meal to help relax the stomach and stimulate it into producing enough enzymes and digestive juices. He was able to do this discreetly during meetings, and it brought considerable relief. He also cut out orange juice from his diet and reduced his alcohol intake considerably. When he came back for a reflexology treatment, as his digestive problems had returned, I taught him the synergistic hand techniques and showed him how to work the stomach reflex on the top of his standing foot when placed on a chair. He was delighted with the results and felt he was getting back in control of the situation again. He told me he now regularly uses VRT as a preventative measure and works the digestive reflexes on his foot after breakfast in the kitchen and after lunch in the office.

reflexology, the more you will know what suits you and what constitutes a good session. This in turn makes you more sensitive to the needs of others who come for a treatment. Gradually introduce certain reflexology skills and techniques that you have enjoyed into your own practice, and keep experimenting on your own feet.

Treating yourself will no longer be a sterile experience. By working your hands and feet simultaneously, preferably while weight-bearing, you will gain the same extra VRT benefits you give to others. One reflexologist who learnt some VRT Synergistic self-help techniques said that working on his own feet had now 'become a dialogue between myself and my body, rather than just pressing the reflexes and asking if there was anybody there'.

Vertical Reflex Therapy Self-help Hand Crib Sheet

Do not treat the hands with VRT for more than five minutes maximum in any one session. Often two or three minutes is all that is required to obtain results.

VRT self-help hand treatment step by step

With self-help techniques you can work one weight-bearing hand completely before starting on the second.

1. Stand in front of a table and firmly place your hand palm downwards. Make sure your arm is straight. For continuity we will start with the right hand.
2. Lean on your arm slightly so that it becomes weight-bearing.
3. Slide/work/brush your thumb across the wrist band several times.
4. **a** 'Banana' – Place your index and third finger under your palm where the thenar muscle is situated (below the base of the thumb) and grip the palm and pull gently upwards three times to work the spinal reflexes.

   b Spinal reflexes – Press vertebrae reflexes from tip of thumb to your wrist with your thumb, index finger or four fingers. Work the reflexes three times.

   c Tap up and down on the spinal reflexes of the hand three times.
5. Pinch round the mid point of your arm between the elbow and the wrist to work the thoracic reflexes.
6. Work your thumb and then fingers with a rotating movement along the top, from nail to base, and make a pinching movement down the side of each finger and the thumb.
7. Press lymphatic reflexes at the base of all the fingers in a rotating movement.
8. Return, at least once, to the wrist points to energise the body.
9. Press ovary/testes helper reflex at the base of the palm in the centre of the hand.
10. Metacarpals (top of the hand) – Work down with four fingers from the wrist band to the fingertips three times.

To conclude:

11. Pituitary Pinch – Pinch thumb firmly for thirty seconds with the nail of your index finger on the table and the tip of your thumb pressing on your thumb nail.

Now repeat moves 1–11 on the other hand.

Key points to remember

1. Self-help reflexology has always enhanced professional treatments and assists the body between sessions.
2. Do not look on self-help VRT as a special treat – see it as essential to your well-being.
3. Conventional self-help reflexology requires you to sit in a comfortable chair. Work your feet for as long as possible – up to half an hour or more.
4. Synergistic self-help VRT means you work two reflexes at once – your right hand is on your right foot, and your left hand works your right hand while it works your foot. Easy once you learn!
5. Synergistic VRT self-help can be weight-bearing but gives you the scope to treat yourself while sitting or standing, anywhere and any time. You can work your feet for longer if you sit down but, when standing, work a maximum of three reflexes synergistically for thirty seconds per reflex.
6. Self-help VRT involves standing firmly with one foot on a wooden chair or stool. Lean on the foot for extra weight-bearing.
7. Do not underestimate self-help VRT Hand Reflexology. It is a very accessible treatment, the hand can easily bear weight on a table, and you can even soothe yourself to sleep with Diaphragm Rocking.
8. Teach your clients and friends these self-help techniques and they will be able to enhance your treatments between sessions.
9. Listen to your body. If your back is aching and you can't stand up, work your weight-bearing hands on a stool beside your chair or sit and work your feet synergistically. Be flexible in your approach.
10. The most important advice is to limit your weight-bearing self-help to a total of five minutes per treatment. Any longer is unnecessary and can overstimulate the body's healing response.

Guide to treating common ailments with VRT

VRT AND REFLEXOLOGY ARE NOT ALTERNATIVE THERAPIES BUT AN ADDITIONAL benefit in the quest for good health. The suggested reflexes listed on p. 173 for treating common ailments should never replace prescribed medicine or treatment without prior consultation with your doctor. Reflexology is an holistic treatment and Basic VRT will treat the entire body. The areas of weakness in the body are sometimes in need of a little more focused reflex stimulation and the charts will help you decide where to work. They are not definitive, so be flexible in your approach and be guided by the information from the client or the tenderness of the reflexes. When you have gained more experience you will be able to select for yourself the most important reflexes to work synergistically and with the Zonal Triggers.

Consult your doctor at once if you have any undiagnosed illness, pain or bleeding. Look also at the list of contra-indications for VRT on pp. 67–9.

Your questions answered

'I know testicular cancer can be a killer, even in young men. I check regularly for any signs such as lumps, but can VRT offer extra help?'

One of the best forms of preventative medicine is to have your body regularly balanced with VRT and conventional reflexology. In between, a five-minute weekly self-help treatment is a good idea. Pay special attention in this instance to the original testes reflex on the outer side of the ankle, and to the helper testes point at the base of the heel. If possible, also have a professional reflexology treatment every month to maintain balance. If you do suspect changes in your testicles, consult your doctor straightaway.

'I have had no interest in sex since the menopause. Can VRT or conventional reflexology help?'

The hormonal balancing effect of all reflexology treatments will certainly be of use here. It is, however, a myth that working the sexual organ reflexes can actually produce sexual arousal. What stimulating these reflexes does is to help balance the body and clear the zones, so that the natural human responses can be turned on when the stimulus is appropriate. Before going to bed couples can share a simple treatment, starting with VRT at the beginning only, with the emphasis on the reproductive organs, the hormones and the brain and spinal reflexes. After this they should lie down and give each other the relaxation techniques and Diaphragm Rocking. Pressing the reflexes on the sole with the thumbs can help the body become more energised. But also look to your general health and stress levels. If after a few weeks, VRT has no effect, maybe you need to explore other sources of help for emotional and physical problems.

> Constipation and irritable bowel are some of the most common ailments in Western society, and reflexology has a positive role to play here. On 24 June 1992 the *Danish Journal of Nursing* reported a careful study of the effects of fifteen weekly half-hour reflexology treatments on twenty women between the ages of thirty and sixty who had suffered from constipation for an average of 24.6 years. All reported an improvement of bowel function, with the average interval between bowel actions reduced from 4.1 to 1.8 days. In addition, 85 per cent reported a positive change in their digestion and 55 per cent were able to reduce their use of laxatives.

'How can VRT help with infertility problems?'

Reflexology and VRT are excellent at stimulating the hormonal system and reproductive organs. If infertility is a problem I work the feet with VRT at the beginning and end of a session and concentrate on the Zonal Triggers for the ovaries. It is important to apply VRT on one of the two peak days for ovulation, so therapist and client need to keep in close touch. In several cases my colleagues and I vigorously worked both ovary reflexes with ZT and held the reflexes on each ankle for thirty to forty-five seconds. Four women treated thus became pregnant after trying unsuccessfully for years. There is no proof that VRT can claim the credit, but the technique is so short and simple that it is always worth trying.

'Is it safe even for a professional reflexologist to work on a woman who is receiving IVF treatment to assist conception?'

Yes. Work the reproductive and all other glands regularly during the months leading up to the IVF treatment. I believe that reflexology complements all allopathic treatments. Once impregnation has taken place I continue to give gentle reflexology treatments with a minute of VRT at the beginning and end of each session, though I brush rather than press the reproductive reflexes. At four months I introduce gentle VRT to the reproductive reflexes.

'I am only in my early forties but often fail to maintain, or even get, an erection. Could VRT help?'

Gentle reflexology can often help correct impotence without the need for medication or counselling, but do consult your doctor if you feel you may have a health problem. The main reflexes to work are the glands, reproductive organs and genitalia. Basic VRT treatment should be followed by work on the lower spinal reflexes, brain and reproductive organs. For up to four weeks your partner should give you two or three minutes of VRT before you get into bed, followed by Diaphragm Rocking. Do not attempt to have sex for at least two weeks – if you fail, the disappointment will only make matters worse. Give your body time to relax and respond, during which your anticipation will increase.

How to use this chart

This reference chart can be used for all three types of VRT treatments: Five-minute Basic, Complete VRT or as part of a full reflexology treatment.

1. Select the condition and work the entire foot in the usual way using Basic VRT, but briefly concentrate on the areas in the column headed 'Main reflexes to be worked'. During the conventional part of the treatment you can return to work these priority areas several times on the reclining feet.
2. At the end of a treatment, whether it lasts two or three minutes or an hour, return to the reflexes of the ankle on the standing feet. Work the ankles and brush across the Zonal Triggers.
3. Select the two synergistic reflexes listed and work the corresponding hand and foot reflexes at the same time. Repeat on the other foot.
4. Select the priority reflex on the top of the foot and hold. Work round the bracelet of the ankle carefully until you locate the relevant Zonal Trigger. Link the reflex and ZT with one of your hands, and find the corresponding reflex on the client's hand. Hold all three for thirty seconds, then repeat on the other foot.
5. Diaphragm Rocking should, ideally, be used after every treatment including five-minute Basic VRT, and fifteen rocks per foot should be the minimum. In some cases, it is appropriate to rock the feet for much longer (up to four minutes in total) to allow the energy to be pumped to the priority area in the body. These instructions are given in the column headed 'Zonal Triggers'.
6. Advanced techniques can be added to the treatment at your discretion. Follow the guidelines in Chapter 8.
7. Remember that Basic VRT can take up to five minutes, but usually takes less. If you intend to use advanced techniques in any one session, keep the Basic VRT moves to a minimum to allow two or three minutes for specialised techniques.

Condition	Main reflexes to be worked	Synergistic reflexes	Zonal Triggers
Acne	Liver, all glands, colon, kidneys	Adrenals/colon	Liver
AIDS/HIV	Liver, all glands, lymphatics, areas most affected	Area most affected, lymphatics	Liver
Alcoholism	Liver, pancreas, diaphragm, brain, solar plexus	Brain/pancreas	Liver DR 3 mins
Allergies	Adrenals, ovaries/testes, areas most affected	Adrenals, ovaries/testes	Area most affected
Anaemia	Spleen, liver	Liver	Spleen
Angina	Heart (ankle reflex), heart/lung, diaphragm, sigmoid colon, thoracic calf points	Sigmoid colon/ diaphragm	Heart/helper reflex DR 2 mins
Arthritis	Entire foot, spine, adrenals, kidneys, areas most affected	Spine, adrenals	Area most affected
Asthma	Diaphragm, chest/lung, bronchi, ileocecal valve, adrenals	Bronchi, adrenals	Chest/lung DR 2–3 mins
Backache	Full spine, neck/shoulder, pelvic/sciatic	Pelvic/sciatic, neck	Appropriate spinal reflex
Bedwetting	Whole spine, diaphragm, bladder, adrenals, brain	Bladder/brain	Lumbar spine DR 2 mins
Cataracts	Eyes/ears, pituitary gland, cervical spine, kidneys	Cervical spine, kidneys	Ears/eyes
Colds and flu	Solar plexus, diaphragm, chest/lung, bronchi, ileocecal valve, adrenals, thyroid gland, lymphatics, ears/eyes	Bronchi, solar plexus	Lymphatics DR 2 mins
Constipation	Colon, liver and gall bladder, adrenals, ileocecal valve, lumbar spine	Lumbar spine, liver	Colon DR 2 mins
Coughs	Chest/lung, throat, lymphatics	Throat, chest/lung	Lymphatics
Cystitis	Bladder, kidneys, ureters, lumbar spine, adrenals	Lumbar spine, ureters	Bladder
Depression	Solar plexus, diaphragm, pituitary, neck, adrenals, brain (work all toes)	Solar plexus, pituitary	Brain DR 2 mins
Diabetes	Pancreas, all glands, liver	Liver, thyroid	Pancreas
Diarrhoea	Small intestine, colon, lumbar spine, solar plexus, ileocecal valve, liver, adrenals	Lumbar spine, liver	Colon
Drug addiction	Solar plexus, diaphragm, adrenals, thyroid, pituitary, brain, liver, kidneys (work all toes)	Liver, kidneys	Brain DR 3 mins
Earache	All toes, cervical spine, eyes/ears, adrenals	Adrenals, cervical spine	Eyes/ears
Eczema	Lymphatics, adrenals, intestines, kidneys, solar plexus, pituitary, areas most affected	Area most affected, kidneys	Lymphatics DR 3 mins
Eye problems	Ears/eyes, kidneys, cranial nerves, neck (work all toes)	Cervical spine, kidneys	Ears/eyes
Fainting	Heart, brain, pituitary, cervical spine	Heart, brain	Pituitary
Fatigue	Diaphragm, solar plexus, heart, all glands, brain, spleen, spine, adrenals	Pituitary, adrenals	Solar plexus DR 2–3 mins
Fever	Pituitary, thyroid, cervical spine	Thyroid, cervical spine	Pituitary
Flatulence	Sigmoid colon, intestines, stomach, solar plexus	Stomach, solar plexus	Intestines

Condition	Main reflexes to be worked	Synergistic reflexes	Zonal Triggers
Gall stones	Liver and gall bladder, thyroid, solar plexus, diaphragm	Thyroid, liver	Gall bladder
Glandular fever	Lymphatics, spleen, pituitary, diaphragm, solar plexus, areas most affected e.g. glands or neck	Areas most affected, pituitary	Lymphatics
Haemorrhoids	Colon, lumbar spine, rectum	Colon, lumbar spine	Rectum
Hangover	Liver, head/brain, kidney	Head/brain, kidney	Liver DR 2 mins
Hay fever	Head, throat, sinuses, eyes, adrenals	Adrenals, throat	Sinuses
Headache	Head, cervical and lumbar spine, solar plexus, intestines, liver	Cervical spine, intestines	Head DR 2–3 mins
Heartburn/ Indigestion	Diaphragm, stomach, solar plexus, oesophagus	Diaphragm, oesophagus	Stomach DR 2 mins
Hernia (abdominal)	Colon, groin, adrenals, spinal reflexes	Adrenals, colon	Groin
Hiatus hernia	Diaphragm, adrenals, stomach, chest/lung	Diaphragm, adrenals	Stomach
Hip problems	Lumbar spine, hip/knee, sciatic, shoulder (referred pain link)	Sciatic, lumbar spine	Hip/knee
Hypertension (high blood pressure)	Kidneys, diaphragm, solar plexus, all glands, heart	Kidneys, heart	Diaphragm DR 2 mins
Hypotension (low blood pressure)	Diaphragm, solar plexus, all glands, heart, thyroid, kidneys	Kidneys, heart	Diaphragm DR 2 mins
Impotence	All glands, reproductive organs, spinal reflexes, diaphragm, brain	Brain, reproductive organs	Testes DR 3 mins
Incontinence	Bladder, kidneys, ureters, lumbar spine, solar plexus, diaphragm	Lumbar spine, solar plexus	Ureter/bladder
Infertility	All glands, diaphragm, solar plexus, lumbar spine, brain, uterus	Thyroid, lumbar spine	Ovary DR 3 mins
Insomnia	All toes, cervical spine, neck, shoulder, pituitary/pineal gland, solar plexus, brain	Solar plexus, pituitary/pineal	Brain DR 3–4 mins
Irritable bowel	Intestines, solar plexus, diaphragm, adrenals, lumbar spine, liver	Lumbar spine adrenals	Colon
Jet lag	Diaphragm, hypothalamus, neck, brain, solar plexus	Brain, neck	Hypothalamus DR 3 mins
Kidney stones	Adrenals, ureters, kidney	Adrenals, ureters	Kidneys
Knee problems	Hip/knee reflexes, lumbar spine, sciatic. Work the elbow (referral area)	Lumbar spine, sciatic	Hip/knee reflexes
Lupus	Spinal reflexes, intestines, liver, spleen, all glands, diaphragm	Intestines, spine	Liver
ME (myalgic encephalo-myelitis) and post-viral syndrome	Brush reflexes for maximum 1 min – 30 secs a foot for first three treatments. All glands, lymphatics, spleen, solar plexus/diaphragm, areas most affected, head	Lymphatics, adrenals	Head DR 3–4 mins
Menopause/hot flushes	All glands, diaphragm, solar plexus, kidneys, uterus	Pituitary, uterus	Thyroid
Menstrual pain	Fallopian tubes, lumbar spine, uterus, all glands, diaphragm, solar plexus	Ovary, lumbar spine	Uterus

Condition	Main reflexes to be worked	Synergistic reflexes	Zonal Triggers
Migraine	Head, eyes, stomach, cervical and lumbar spine, solar plexus, intestines,liver, spine	Stomach, cervical spine	Head
Multiple sclerosis	Diaphragm, solar plexus, spine, brain, all glands	Solar plexus, brain	Spine
Neck problems	Neck, cervical spine, lumbar spine, shoulder	Neck, shoulder	Spine
Paralysis	Whole spine, brain, area most affected	Brain, area most affected	Whole spine
PMT	Solar plexus, all glands, affected areas e.g. abdomen or uterus	Pituitary, solar plexus	Area most affected
Pregnancy	Brush all reflexes lightly in first four months. Then work solar plexus, uterus, all glands, bladder, adrenals, lumbar spine	Pituitary, lumbar spine	Solar plexus
Sciatica	Diaphragm, solar plexus, lower lumbar spine, sciatic, shoulder, hip/knee	Lower lumbar spine, hip/knee	Sciatic
Shingles	Lung, chest, lymphatics, affected area, adrenals, pituitary, thyroid, spinal nerves	Lymphatics, thyroid	Affected area
Shoulder problems	Shoulder, arm, thoracic spine, diaphragm, hip	Hip, thoracic spine	Shoulder
Sickness and travel sickness	Stomach, adrenals, head, thoracic spine, lymphatics, ears	Ears, lymphatics	Stomach
Skin problems	Solar plexus, diaphragm, intestines, thyroid, kidneys, pituitary, affected area	Thyroid, solar plexus	Intestines DR 2 mins
Sore throat	Throat/neck, lymphatics, adrenals, solar plexus	Lymphatics	Throat/neck
Stress	Diaphragm, solar plexus, adrenals, pituitary, areas most affected	Areas most affected, solar plexus	Adrenals
Stroke	Toes, reflexes to affected areas, whole spine, dorsal ankle reflexes, brain	Affected areas and dorsal ankle reflex	Brain. Work the alternative side from the paralysis more thoroughly
Thyroid (under- or over-active)	Thyroid, pituitary, adrenal, eyes, cervical spine	Pituitary, cervical spine	Thyroid
Tinnitus	Ears, sinuses, cervical spine, diaphragm, solar plexus, adrenals, Eustachian tube	Cervical spine, sinuses	Ears
Tonsillitis	Lymphatics, toes, cervical spine, adrenals tonsils, throat	Lymphatics, cervical spine	Throat – between end of nail and first joint on thumb
Toothache	Toes, below nail of big toe, adrenals, cervical spine	Adrenals, cervical spine	Below nail of big toe
Tumours	Whole spine, all glands, solar plexus, areas most affected	Pituitary, solar plexus	Areas most affected
Ulcers (external)	Diaphragm, solar plexus, lymphatics, areas most affected, adrenals	Lymphatics, solar plexus	Areas most affected
Ulcers (internal)	Stomach, duodenum, diaphragm, solar plexus, lymphatics	Stomach, lymphatics	Duodenum
Urinary incontinence	Lumbar spine, kidneys, bladder, ureters, adrenals, brain	Ureters, lumbar spine	Bladder
Varicose veins (legs)	Liver, heart reflex on dorsal ankle, intestines, adrenals, legs, arm as referral area	Liver, adrenals	Legs
Whiplash	Cervical spine, all toes, adrenals, shoulder, neck	Between big and second toe,shoulder	Cervical spine

Glossary of Terms

Abdominal area – this is situated below the chest from which it is separated by the diaphragm. It contains the digestive organs and excretory organs and is lined by a membrane called the peritoneum.

Acupuncture – an ancient Chinese therapy that treats the body by puncturing it with fine needles on specific *meridian* points to balance and heal by regulating the *life force.* It is the most widely known complementary therapy in the West and is increasingly being used in conventional medical practice.

Acute – a condition having rapid onset (the opposite of *chronic*).

Adrenalin – an important hormone secreted from the medulla (core) of the adrenal gland. It has widespread effects on the muscles, circulation and sugar metabolism.

Allergies – a sensitivity disorder where the body becomes hypersensitive to particular allergens which provoke specific symptoms when encountered. Different allergies affect different tissues and produce localised or widespread effects. These can range from respiratory problems from pollen or house dust, gastro-enteritis, skin irritation to potentially fatal shock.

Allopathic medicine – orthodox medical treatment of diseases by drugs, surgery etc.

Ankle band – the part of the ankle at the base of the leg.

Ankle bracelet – the same area as the *ankle band* but is sometimes used in this book to specifically identify the area where the Zonal Triggers are located.

Antibody – a defensive substance within the organisms of the body that reacts to the presence of disease or toxins.

Arthritis – a generic term for a chronic joint disease characterised by loss of some joint cartilage. Rheumatoid arthritis is an autoimmune disease where the synovial membrane of a joint gradually becomes swollen and inflamed.

Calf – the thick fleshy part of the back of the leg below the knee.

Capillary – a minute blood vessel that connects arteries with the veins

Caterpillar bites –a reflexology term to describe the finger or thumb techniques used to precisely work the reflexes by inching the finger (bent at the first joint) across the reflexes in tiny *bites* so as not to miss any area of the foot or hand. It can also be known as caterpillar walking ; see also *thumb* and *finger walking*.

Cervical – 7 vertebrae bones making up neck region of the spine

Chronic – a condition of long duration (the opposite of *acute*).

Collagen – a fibrous connective tissue containing protein

Contra-indication – means unsuitable and is an indication of when *not* to treat.

Cranial nerves – 12 pairs of nerves that have their roots at the base of the brain and supply parts of the head.

Crib sheet – Basic Instructions in abbreviated form.

Cuboid Notch – a slight indentation on the cuboid bone which is situated on the *lateral* (outside) edge of the foot.

Diaphragm – plays an important part in the mechanism of breathing. It is a strong, thin dome-shaped muscle that separates the thoracic and abdominal cavities

Diaphragm Rocking (DR) The diaphragm is represented as a horizontal line that runs below the ball of the foot. This gentle rocking movement, when properly applied, appears to prioritise conditions most in need of help and pumps energy and relaxation to specific parts of the body. Disruptive sleep patterns improve dramatically and it has proved extremely effective in breaking long-term patterns of ill health. Diaphragm Rocking, along with Zonal Triggers, is one of the two most important techniques in the VRT repertoire.

Digit – finger or toe

Dorsal – referring to the top of the foot

Dorsum – the top of the foot (as opposed to the sole)

Endocrine – refers to the hormonal system of the body. The endocrine or ductless glands control long-term changes in the body. They secrete minute quantities of their hormone directly into the body.

Finger Walking – a standard reflexology technique where the finger is bent at the first joint and *inches* across the foot or hand minutely making contact with the reflexes. *Caterpillar walking* is also a term sometimes used to describe this technique.

Forefinger – the first finger after the thumb. Also known as the *index* finger.

Genitalia – the reproductive organs of the male and female particularly the external parts such as the penis, testicles, labia and clitoris.

Glands – are ductless vessels or structures that are specialised for synthesizing and secreting certain fluids for use in the body or for excretion.

Glucose – is an important source of energy and is one of the constituents of sucrose and starch which supply glucose after digestion. It is stored in the body in the form of *glycogen*.

Glycogen – can be readily broken down into *glucose*. It is stored in the muscles and liver and is the principal form in which carbohydrate is stored in the body.

Healing crisis – is a natural reaction to a complementary treatment which can occasionally result when the body is stimulated to throw off toxins too quickly. This can result in a short period, usually a few hours, of possibly vomiting or bowel disorders, skin sensitivity or increased pain. It can also result in a headache. All these symptoms can often be prevented by asking the client to drink much more water following a treatment. Some practitioners have created a minor healing crisis for their clients by using VRT for up to 15 minutes in a treatment, instead of five, against all good advice. In all reports the person then felt better than ever once the symptoms subsided but the discomfort suffered had been unnecessary. *Side effects* are a milder version of a healing crisis.

Helper reflexes – these specifically refer to the new reflexes discovered in VRT that support, and are linked, to the original reflexes, i.e. the helper heart, ovary and diaphragm reflexes. By working the *helper reflexes* a treatment can be enhanced.

Holistic – an approach to health that aims to treat the person as an entity where the body, mind spirit are assumed to co-exist and are all given consideration.

Homeostasis – a Greek word meaning *a state of balance* or equilibrium

Hypertension – high blood pressure

Hypotension – low blood pressure

Immune System – is a general term for a complex system that enables the body to resist infection and fight disease. This is afforded by the presence of circulating antibodies and white blood cells.

Index finger – the first finger after the thumb. Also known as the *forefinger*.

Knuckle Dusting – a means of working the toes and dorsum (top) of the foot with the knuckles the fist of the hand uses light twisting and sweeping movements. It is extremely powerful in treating conditions as diverse as asthma, depression and irritable bowel. Use for only 15 seconds on each foot.

Lateral – refers to the outside edge of the foot or hand

Libido – the sexual drive. Usually refers to the degree of intensity

Life Force – an energy and innate form of self healing within the body.

Longitudinal Zones – Ten vertical reflexology zones in the body, five on each side and starting on the toes and fingers, that act as conduits for healing and stimulation from *reflex points* to particular parts of the body.

Lumbar – refers to the five lower vertebrae in the back. These are situated between the thoracic vertebrae and the sacrum/coccyx at the base of the spine. The lumbar spine refers to the lower back.

Lymph – Glands – are principally found in the neck, groin and armpits and the small vessels that link them are called lymphatics which contain a thin fluid called *lymph*.

Lymph – is the thin fluid present within the *lymphatic system*. Lymph contains some protein and some cells which are mainly lymphocytes.

Lymphatic system – a network of vessels in the body that carries water, proteins, electrolytes etc in the form of lymph from the tissue fluids to the blood stream.

ME (Myalgic encephalo-myelitis) – a form of post-viral syndrome often following influenza or glandular fever and has many symptoms including chronic tiredness, digestive problems and general lack of energy. Post-viral conditions are usually identified as ME when the patient presents painful, tender muscles. The condition can last for years.

Medial – refers to the inside edge of the foot or hand.

Meridian Lines – a term in acupuncture that describes the channels that run through the body carrying the *life force* or *chi*. There are 14 main meridians in Chinese acupuncture that run from the hands and feet to the body and the head.

Metabolism – is the collection of all the chemical and physical changes that take place within the body. It is the process by which the body grows and functions.

Metatarsal Pressure – an advanced VRT weight-bearing technique where the foot is highly arched with all pressure on the ball of the foot. The back, shoulder and neck reflexes become much more responsive in this position.

Metacarpals – the longest bones in the hands. They connect to the *phalanges* (finger bones)

Metatarsals – longest bones in the feet. They connect to the *phalanges* (toe bones)

Navicular bone – the boat-shaped bone of the ankle that articulates with the three cuniform bones and the talus bone behind.

Nerve Pathways – same meaning as *neural pathways* which denote the complex system of 31 pairs of spinal nerves that emanate from the spinal cord to various parts of the body and relay messages to and from the brain.

Nervous System – Autonomic – supplies all the body structures over which we have no control. It is divided into two separate parts – the sympathetic and parasympathetic systems.

Neural Pathway reflexes – are situated in the same area as the spinal reflexes which run down the medial edge of the foot and hand (inside edge) – being the primary set of spinal reflexes. The term *neural pathways* refers to the 31 pairs of nerves which emanate from the central nervous system (CNS) to various parts of the body and relay messages to and from the brain. The *spinal cord* is protected by the vertebrae that make up the spinal column

Oedema – excessive accumulation of fluid in the body tissues. Subcutaneous oedema commonly occurs in the legs and ankles. Reflexologists should work very gently on swollen feet or work the hands instead.

Orthopaedic – preventative and corrective treatment of the skeletal system.

Osteopathy – is a gentle manipulation of the muscular-skeletal system to realign the framework of the body so that it interacts efficiently with the nervous, circulatory and other systems.

Osteoporosis – loss of bony tissue resulting in fragile and brittle bones. More common in elderly women and can accelerate after the menopause.

Palming – a gentle VRT technique where the heel of the palm is applied to the dorsum of the foot in firm pressing and sweeping movements.

Phalanges – the finger and toe bones.

Pituitary gland – the master gland of the endocrine system. It is a pea-sized body attached to the hypothalamus at the base of the skull. It controls the function of all other glands in the body.

Pituitary Pinch – this is a very powerful VRT technique where the pituitary reflexes (master gland of the endocrine system) on the big toes are simultaneously stimulated when the client is standing.

Plantar – the sole of the foot

Plantar Stepping – an advanced VRT weight-bearing technique where pressure is placed on the ball of the foot while at a 45 degree angle. This enables access to some *plantar* (sole) reflexes at the same time.

Points – in this book it is simply another word for *reflexes*.

Post-viral Syndrome – often follows influenza or glandular fever and has many symptoms including chronic tiredness, digestive problems and a general lack of energy. Post-viral conditions are usually identified as ME (Myalgic encephalo-myelitis) only when the patient presents painful, tender muscles and the condition has been present for many months .

Pre-menstrual Tension (PMT) – a collection of symptoms including bloating, depression, irritability and inability to concentrate that usually occur during the week preceding menstruation.

Referral areas – are useful as an extra tool in reflexology when you want to treat a painful right ankle for example. You would work the right wrist instead. The basic rule is as follows: always link limbs on the same side of the body i.e. right to right: *hip* links with *shoulder, thigh* links with *upper arm, elbow* links with *knee, calf* links with *forearm, ankle* links with *wrist* and *hand* links with *foot.*

Referred pain – a pain in the body in an area other than the source. This is because the sensory nerves share common pathways to the spinal cord and the brain.

Reflexes are sensitive minute *points* on the feet that are connected to specific parts of the body and can sometimes feel quite tender if they correspond to a malfunctioning part of the body. However, painful areas of the feet do not always indicate ill health, they can simply show vitality! Reflexes can also become tender due to a physical problem on the foot itself, which is totally unconnected with reflexology, and you must be aware of this possibility when treating clients. A reflexologist is trained to detect the difference but the golden rule for everyone is to ease off a painful reflex and work it more gently.

Reflexology is an ancient natural therapy that describes a healing energy that flows from hundreds of specific reflexes in the feet and these reflexes correspond to all the organs, glands and parts of the skeletal system in the body. By gently stimulating certain points with fingers and thumbs, the body itself responds to bring about self-healing and *homeostasis* (the Greek word for 'balance').

Rotating Movement – this refers to a standard reflexology technique where the finger or thumb is placed firmly on a reflex point and rotated in small circular movements to stimulate an energetic response in a particular part of the body.

Sciatic Nerve – it is the major nerve in the leg and runs from the lower end of the spine down the leg to below the thigh.

Sebaceous glands – open into the hair follicles. They are simple or branched glands in the skin that secrete an oily substance called sebum.

Self-help VRT Techniques are essential to the well-being of all therapists and carers and it is a form of instant first-aid that can be applied anywhere. The synergistic approach to self-help is very powerful and you can even work your own foot and hand at the same time.

Senses – sight, hearing, smell, taste and touch are the faculties by which the external world is appreciated.

Side effects – in the context of complementary therapies, they are mild natural reactions to a treatment which can occasionally result when the body is stimulated to throw off toxins, unlike a *healing crisis*, which is a stronger reaction. This can result in a feeling of nausea, headache, greater voiding of urine or faeces but passes within minutes or hours.

Spinal cord – supplies 31 pairs of extremely complex nerves that branch off along the spinal cord to various parts of the body. Reflexologists refer to these in a simplified form when working the *neural or nerve pathways reflexes.*

Steroid – a group of organic hormones that include male and female sex hormones plus the hormones of the adrenal cortex. Synthetic replacement hormones are manufactured for medical purposes.

Synergistic – combined or co-ordinated actions that, when used together, increases the effect of the other. In VRT the simultaneous working of the hand and foot reflexes greatly increases the response of the body as opposed to working each reflex separately.

Synergistic Reflexology (SR) is a VRT technique where hand and foot reflexes are worked simultaneously. This technique can accelerate the body's response and, in orthopaedic cases, increased mobility has sometimes been achieved in minutes. SR also works when the client is lying or sitting down and the person being treated can be taught to work their own appropriate hand reflexes.

Systems of the body – these comprise various groups of organs, glands, nerves and skeletal structures, each of which performs a specific function. The systems of the body are interdependent on each other.

Tendon – a tough band of fibrous tissue forming the end of a muscle and attached to the bone. Reflexologists should take care not to exert undue pressure on the tendon on the *medial* (inside) sole of the foot. No pressure at all should be placed on the tendon when the foot is weight-bearing as in *Plantar Stepping and Metatarsal Pressure*.

Thigh – the upper part of the leg between the hip and the knee.

Thoracic – refers to 12 bones of the backbone or spine to which the ribs are attached. They are situated between the *cervical* and *lumbar* vertebrae.

Thumb Walking – a standard reflexology technique where the thumb is bent at the first joint and *inches* across the foot or hand minutely making contact with the reflexes. *Caterpillar walking* is also a term sometimes used to describe this technique.

Toxins – A poison produced by living organisms in the body, especially bacteria.

Transverse Zones – are horizontal lines on the foot that mark the shoulder girdle, waistline and pelvic floor position and the relative position of the reflexes on the foot.

Tuberosity – Protuberance on a bone

Varicose veins – these can be fine or thick veins that are distorted, lengthened and tortuous. The most common site is in the legs. Many fine varicose veins can cover the feet.

Vertebra (plural *vertebrae*) – one of the 33 bones, including the sacrum/coccyx, that comprise the spine or backbone. The arch of each vertebra contains part of the spinal cord. Vertebrae are bound together by ligaments and intervertebral discs.

Vertical Reflex Therapy (VRT) is the overall term for this new form of reflexology which treats the dorsum (top) of the foot while in standing position. The foot reflexes become far more sensitive and responsive to pressure when weight-bearing.

Zonal Triggers (ZT) are deep VRT reflex points on the ankles that appear to accelerate the healing to deep-seated problems in the body when linked to two specific reflexes. They are simple to detect and use and are, along with Diaphragm Rocking, one of the two most important techniques in the VRT repertoire.

Zones – are ten longitudinal energetic reflexology lines which run throughout the body starting at the fingers and the toes – five on each side. The flow of energy affects and stimulates all parts of the body situated within each zone. Reflexology acts as a stimulus to remove blocks in the zones that can create ill-health and inhibit the *life force*.

Finding a therapist

It is very important that you find the right therapist of whatever calling. People are often baffled by the range on offer, and there are few regulations about who can practise complementary therapies. Most complementary practitioners belong to organisations that represent their interests and regulate standards in practice and training. But many members of the public are unable to ascertain whether an official-looking certificate on a therapist's wall means they are qualified to give a full professional treatment or only attended a weekend course for beginners. An additional problem is that bona fide practitioners may undertake full professional training in one therapy and then explore others via short weekend courses. The danger comes when an efficient practitioner in a particular therapy offers themselves as an expert in another field of complementary medicine in which they have had only minimal training. So how can you avoid these pitfalls and enjoy the degree of expert care and attention you deserve?

When seeking a practitioner it is often helpful to speak to more than one, to see if they answer your questions helpfully. Word of mouth is one of the best recommendations. It is important that you feel comfortable with them. Most reflexologists expect to treat someone once or possibly twice a week for four to six sessions, and then assess progress. But some people expect immediate results, especially if they have heard about some of the successes with VRT. Be fair on the practitioner – be prepared to give your body time to make some fundamental health changes.

The following guidelines will ensure success in finding a good practitioner. A dedicated and professional therapist will be not in the least offended by you asking questions. Fully qualified reflexologists and complementary therapists in general are equally concerned about the current lack of regulation within their chosen profession.

Before booking an appointment with a complementary therapist ask the following questions:

- Are they a full member of a professional organisation that regulates the therapy they are advertising?

- How long have they been qualified, and which school or institute did they train with?
- How long was their training?
- Are they fully insured?

If you want to know of a qualified practitioner in your area, then telephone an appropriate organisation from those listed overleaf. Alternatively look for a wider list of complementary regulatory bodies in health magazines such as *Positive Health* and *Here's Health*, which are sold in newsagents throughout the country. Some professional organisations or institutes place block advertisements in the *Yellow Pages* advertising their members in a particular region.

Reflexology training

I hope this book will not only have encouraged people to experience some reflexology sessions for the first time, but will also have inspired some to investigate the possibilities of training to be a reflexologist themselves. There are many schools of reflexology and technical colleges that offer comprehensive training. Study times vary, and there are courses run on weekdays, evenings or weekends. It is important to shop around, study prospectuses and talk to the tutors. The amount of time and money spent on training makes a reflexology course a big investment, and you need to feel comfortable and positive about all aspects of it. The outcome should be a professional qualification, and the confidence to start a new and fulfilling career. Groundwork is essential. The Association of Reflexologists is the largest reflexology body and can supply a list of accredited schools in your area. If you are already qualified as a reflexologist there are many postgraduate courses and workshops to help further your knowledge, and most reflexology bodies make it a requirement of membership that their graduates undertake further study every year or so to keep up with developments.

Useful Addresses

Booth VRT
Suite 205
60 Westbury Hill
Westbury-on-Trym
Bristol
BS9 3UJ
Email: boothvrt@waitrose.com
Website:www.boothvrt.co.uk

Vertical Reflex Therapy courses are run for qualified reflexologists throughout the UK and internationally exclusively by Lynne Booth and VRT Appointed Tutors. For details about VRT in general, course venue information and telephone numbers of trained VRT practitioners in specific areas, please send a stamped addressed envelope to the above address stating your requirement.

Advanced Reflexology Training (ART)
Director: Anthony Porter
28 Hollyfield Avenue
London
N11 3BY
Tel: 0208 368 0865
Fax 0208 368 1269
E-mail: artreflex@btinternet.com
Website:www.artreflex.com

ART courses are run in the UK and internationally for qualified reflexologists. Anthony Porter has developed many exceptional techniques that can produce a powerful response to the body's inherent healing potential. He has published an authoritative book on the practice and philosophy of ART techniques, obtainable from the above address. ART techniques can enhance Vertical Reflex Therapy for the practitioner.

Association of Reflexologists
27 Old Gloucester Street
London
WC1N 3XX
Tel: 0870 5673320
Website:www.reflexology.org/aor

The Association is an independent organisation and aims to maintain high standards of practice. Members of the public, who want to consult a reliable practitioner, can request a Referral Register. The Association also publishes a list of schools and training establishments, for those wishing to train in reflexology, that meet the level for accreditation.

International Institute of Reflexology
Head Office (UK)
Hill House
255 Turleigh
Bradford-on-Avon
Wiltshire
BA15 2HG
Tel/Fax: 01225 865899

The International Institute was started by the founder of modern reflexology, Eunice Ingham, and is dedicated to maintaining professional standards in reflexology training. Highly professional courses are taught throughout the world under the auspices of the President, Dwight Byers, who is Ingham's nephew. The IIR is accredited by the Open and Distance Learning Quality Control Council for its overall standard of service to students.

Kristine Walker Hand Reflexology
223 Hartington Road
Brighton
BN2 3PA

Kristine Walker has been a remarkable influence on Hand Reflexology and has increased reflexologists' awareness that the healing potential of reflexology is as great in the hands as in the feet. Her book *Hand Reflexology* is also a very useful reference text when using VRT synergistically.

Institute for Complementary Medicine
PO Box 194
London
SE16 1QZ
Tel: 0207 237 5765

The ICM is a charity that aims to offer the public an informed choice of safe Complementary Medicine practised by professionals trained to a high standard of competence. Members must satisfy the institute that they adhere to the Code of Ethics and fulfil all membership criteria. ICM publish the British Register of Complementary Practitioners.

Institute for Optimum Nutrition (ION)
Blades Court
Deodar Road
London
SW15 2NU
Tel: 0208 877 9993

High standard of training for nutritionists. Can provide names of qualified practitioners.

Bristol Cancer Help Centre
Grove House
Cornwallis Grove
Clifton
Bristol
BS8 4PG
Tel: 0117 980 9500
Helpline: 0117 980 9505
Fax: 0117 923 9184
Website: www.bristolcancerhelp.org

Residential courses: The Centre offers a fully integrated programme of self-help techniques which work alongside medical treatments to promote positive health, fighting spirit and psychological well-being in those with cancer and their supporters.

HELP
2B North Way
Bounds Green Industrial Estate
Bounds Green
London N11 2UL
Tel: 0208 361 9984
Fax: 0208 361 2815

Suppliers of the Porta-ped mini couch for reflexologists and chiropodists, which is portable and provides a stable foot rest at the right height for both practitioner and client.

Recommended reading

Batmanghelidj, Dr F. *Your Body's Many Cries for Water* Tagman Press (2000)

Carroll, Steve, *The Which? Guide to Men's Health* Penguin Books (1999)

Holford, Patrick, *The Optimum Nutrition Bible* Piatkus Books (1998)

Marsden, Kathryn, *The Complete Book of Food Combining* Piatkus Books (2000)

Norman, Laura, *The Reflexology Handbook* Piatkus Books (1989)

Shealey, Norman C. (ed), *The Complete Family Guide to Alternative Medicine* Element Books (1999)

Smith, Karen, *Body and Soul – a Woman's Guide to Staying Young* Kyle Cathie Ltd (1997)

Walker, Kristine, *Hand Reflexology* Quay Books (1996)

de Vries, Jan, *The Five Senses* Mainstream Publishing (1997)

Monthly publications which cover complementary health topics

Positive Health (tel: 0117 983 8851). Subscription or from newsagents/ health shops

Here's Health (tel: 01858 438869). Subscription or from newsagents/ health shops

Journal of Alternative and Complementary Medicine (tel: 0207 385 0012). Subscription

What Doctors Don't Tell You (tel: 0207 354 4592). Subscription

Medical Trial of Complete VRT

Complete VRT was not as complete as it is now when I conducted a small medical trial at the St Monica residential nursing home in Bristol in June 1997, although the overall results were still very positive. I was then using Synergistic Reflexology and Zonal Triggers in a very experimental way, and decided not to include them in the shortened trial treatments. Each resident who took part was given a fifteen-minute treatment of three minutes' VRT at the beginning, conventional reflexology while they reclined on a couch, and then another two minutes of VRT. In the published results over 60 per cent of the residents reported improvement, including two cases where a major breakthrough in recovery seemed to occur. Two months later the improvements in all cases appeared to be sustained.

St Monica Home is one of the largest residential homes in the West of England and offers accommodation for nearly two hundred residents in sheltered accommodation and full nursing care. I reasoned that a medical trial would be a useful method of proving the efficacy of VRT before I wrote a paper on the subject for my professional body, as many residents, as well as medical and administrative staff, had been benefiting from Vertical Reflex Therapy in my weekly clinics there.

Seven residents, who had never had reflexology before, were put forward by the Matron. All had a multiplicity of health problems but the common factor was lack of mobility in hips, knees and back. It was not my intention to treat specific ailments but simply to reassess the individual's condition after six weeks to ascertain whether there was any increase in mobility and decrease in pain.

First I took a case history and explained the concept of reflexology to each participant and gave them a brief introductory treatment lasting about a minute. Interestingly, the six-week trial had to be written up as a seven-week trial because the diaries, which were authenticated by the medical staff, indicated that two improvements to an arm and a neck had occurred after the initial one-minute VRT treatment!

Ninety-year-old Mrs H, however, reacted badly to her first session: she had neck pains and fatigue and felt very emotional, so she decided to withdraw from the study. I then invited Mr V to replace her, as he had a long-standing hip problem.

The two most successful results illustrated the wide-ranging benefits of VRT. Mrs A, seventy-three, began walking round her room unaided for the first time in a year and had less shoulder and neck pain. Her great joy was to brush her hair easily again and shake off an undefined 'tenderness on her skin and emotional depression'. Mrs B, sixty-one, gained enormous benefits from VRT. A permanent excruciating groin pain dissipated in three treatments – although her knee problem failed to respond to VRT at all. Her painful groin reflex could only be located when she was standing.

Others, like Mr V, found they could walk much better with less hip pain, although it was not until after the trial was over that he became fully aware of his new mobility and increased walking power. This was unfortunate, as he was recorded as a failure in the statistics. Two months later he became the first person to regain flexibility in his hip thanks to Synergistic Reflexology.

The trial's findings were evaluated on the increase in mobility over the seven-week period, but other aspects of improvement included one lady becoming much calmer and reporting that she had had no temper outbursts for seven weeks, which apparently was something of a record! Another person stated that her back was a little better but she had suffered a debilitating headache after each VRT session. The last time she had experienced such a headache was forty years previously during a very traumatic time when she first had to wear a heavy National Health wig during a heatwave. She bravely kept coming for all the treatments, as she felt her back was improving and she wanted to help with the trial.

The trial was a landmark in the development of VRT. All the participants were medically monitored at all times and their progress, or otherwise, was recorded with the help of medical staff and cooperation from the GPs involved. The trial results, when published, encouraged many reflexologists to experiment with these unique weight-bearing techniques. It was reasonable to assume that, if VRT could work so well on the chronically sick and elderly, it could work well on anyone.

Index